Psychology Revivals

Cancer, Nutrition, and Eating Behavior

The majority of cancer-related deaths are associated with nutritional problems. The major role that nutrition and diet play in the development and course of cancer had only been recently appreciated, and relatively little had been written on the topic in general. A critical component of nutrition and diet is eating behavior. Originally published in 1985, the purpose of this book was to meet the needs of both the clinician and the researcher by bringing together data and theory about nutrition and cancer from several disciplines, as considered from a biobehavioral perspective.

The first chapter of the book provides an overview of the purposes and organization of the volume. The rest is divided into 3 parts. Part 1 focuses on basic research concerned with the nature and development of taste aversions and taste preferences in human and animals. Part 2 applies the basic processes reviews in the first part to the cancer area, focusing on eating and nutritional problems related to both tumor development and to learned processes that develop as a result of being exposed to radiotherapy and chemotherapy treatments. Part 3 focuses on identifying and evaluating intervention strategies for improving the nutritional status of people with cancer or at high risk for developing cancer.

Cancer, Nutrition, and Eating Behavior

A Biobehavioral Perspective

Edited by
Thomas G. Burish, Sandra M. Levy
and Beth E. Meyerowitz

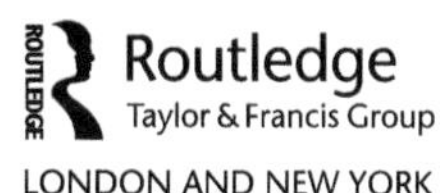

LONDON AND NEW YORK

First published in 1985
by Lawrence Erlbaum Associates, Inc.

This edition first published in 2021 by Routledge
2 Park Square, Milton Park, Abingdon, Oxon OX14 4RN

and by Routledge
605 Third Avenue, New York, NY 10017

Routledge is an imprint of the Taylor & Francis Group, an informa business

Publisher's Note
The publisher has gone to great lengths to ensure the quality of this reprint but points out that some imperfections in the original copies may be apparent.

Disclaimer
The publisher has made every effort to trace copyright holders and welcomes correspondence from those they have been unable to contact.

A Library of Congress record exists under ISBN: 0898595185

ISBN 13: 978-0-367-62127-8 (pbk)
ISBN 13: 978-0-367-62086-8 (hbk)
ISBN 13: 978-1-003-10803-0 (ebk)

CANCER, NUTRITION, AND EATING BEHAVIOR:

A Biobehavioral Perspective

Edited by

Thomas G. Burish
Vanderbilt University

Sandra M. Levy
University of Pittsburgh Medical School

Beth E. Meyerowitz
Vanderbilt University

LEA LAWRENCE EARLBAUM ASSOCIATES, PUBLISHERS
1985 Hillsdale, New Jersey London

Lawrence Erlbaum Associates, Inc., Publishers
365 Broadway
Hillsdale, New Jersey 07642

Library of Congress Cataloging in Publication Data
Main entry under title:

Cancer, nutrition, and eating behavior.

Based on a conference held at Vanderbilt University in Mar. 1983.
Includes bibliographies and indexes.
1. Cancer—Congresses. 2. Cancer—Nutritional aspects—Congresses. 3. Cancer—Treatment—Complications and sequelae—Congresses. 4. Cancer—Psychological aspects—Congresses. 5. Food habits—Congresses. I. Burish, Thomas G. II. Levy, Sandra M. III. Meyerowitz, Beth E. [DNLM: 1. Diet—congresses. 2. Feeding Behavior—drug effects—congresses. 3. Feeding behavior—radiation effects—congresses. 4. Neoplasms—etiology—congresses. 5. Neoplasms—therapy—congresses. 6. Nutrition Disorders—etiology—congresses. QZ 200 C215363 1983]
RC261.C2736 1985 616.99'4 84-28731
ISBN 0-89859-518-5

Contents

Preface

The majority of cancer-related deaths are associated with nutritional problems. In some cases, these nutritional problems may play a causal or promotional role in the development of cancer. For example, high dietary fat intake has been associated with the development of breast cancer, and low dietary fiber intake, especially in combination with high fat intake, has been associated with colon cancer. In other cases, nutritional problems may be caused by, and lead to a worsening of, the cancer. For example, certain tumor processes may alter taste sensations so as to decrease the attractiveness of many foods, or may alter one's energy metabolism, resulting in energy expenditure that exceeds normal levels. The treatment of cancer can also produce a variety of nutritional problems. For example, both radiation and chemotherapy can cause mouth sores, diarrhea, nausea, and vomiting. Surgical removal of parts of the gastrointestinal tract can make swallowing difficult, cause diarrhea, or decrease the extent to which ingested food is absorbed. Finally, the presence of cancer and the adverse side effects of cancer treatments can result in a variety of general physiological and psychological changes that alter dietary intake. Feelings of malaise, lack of energy, depression, and learned taste aversions can all produce substantial changes in eating behavior.

The major role that nutrition and diet play in the development and course of cancer has only recently been fully appreciated, and relatively little has been written on the topic in general. A critical component of nutrition and diet is eating behavior. Eating is a behavior that is embedded in a social and cultural context. The eating behavior of both healthy individuals and cancer patients is highly affected by cognitive, emotional, and motivational factors. Moreover, behavioral factors can interact with physical and disease-related variables to affect nutrition and diet. The paucity of relevant research and written material is especially notable in the behavioral area.

As a result of the increased awareness of the role of diet and nutrition in cancer, there is a growing need among clinicians for information that can be used to help prevent and/or treat the nutritional problems commonly experienced by cancer patients, such as cachexia, anorexia, learned taste aversions, and conditioned nausea and vomiting. Similarly, there is a steadily growing cadre of researchers from a variety of disciplines who are seeking to acquaint themselves with the data available in the field of cancer and nutrition and to identify the most productive avenues for future research. The purpose of this book is to meet the needs of both the clinician and the researcher by bringing together data and theory about nutrition and cancer from several disciplines, as considered from a biobehavioral perspective.

This volume grew out of an exciting, multidisciplinary conference entitled "Psychobiological Aspects of Conditioned Taste Aversions and Nutritional Problems in Cancer" which was held at Vanderbilt University in March, 1983. This working conference brought together most of the chapter authors for two days of presentations and active discussion. The purpose of the conference was to facilitate the sharing and the development of knowledge relevant to the interface of cancer, nutrition, and eating behavior. Each of the principal authors presented a draft of his or her chapter at the conference, with each of the other authors commenting on the presentation. Following the conference, authors revised their chapters and these revisions were submitted to three or more of the authors/editors for additional review. The present volume is the product of this active, critical, multidisciplinary review process. The book is designed to serve as the major reference volume for both clinicians and researchers, including physicians, psychologists, dietitians, and nurses. In addition, the volume can be used as graduate-level text or supplementary text for courses on behavioral medicine, nutrition, and cancer.

The first chapter of the book provides an overview of the purposes and organization of the volume, and presents several themes that help to integrate the chapters that follow. The remaining chapters are divided into three sections. Section I focuses on basic research concerned with the nature and development of taste aversions and taste preferences in humans and animals. Section II applies the basic processes reviewed in the first section to the cancer area. The chapters in this section focus on eating and nutritional problems related to both tumor development and to learned processes that develop as a result of being exposed to radiotherapy and chemotherapy treatments. Finally, Section III focuses on identifying and evaluating intervention strategies for improving the nutritional status of people with cancer or at high risk for developing cancer. The first chapter in this section describes the nature and extent of nutritional problems in cancer patients while the second chapter, which is primarily methodological in its focus, discusses some promising techniques for assessing dietary intake and its modification in healthy persons and cancer patients. These two chapters provide the necessary context for understanding the rationale for the several intervention strategies that are described in subsequent chapters, including total parenteral nutrition; behavioral interventions; and large scale, preventative, dietary modification programs.

We wish to acknowledge gratefully the support of several people and organizations. The conference that helped to generate this book was funded by multiple sources: a grant from the Levi Strauss Foundation to the Center for the Study of Families and Children of the Vanderbilt Institute for Public Policy Studies, the Vanderbilt University Research Council, and the Vanderbilt University Department of Psychology. John Masters initiated the idea of a conference and a volume, and he worked closely with us as the idea was transformed into reality. His generous support and perspicacious advice were needed and appreciated. Ira Turkat played an active and creative role in helping us to conceptualize the conference and bring it to fruition. Michael Carey and Jan Williams were indispensable as conference coordinators. Trish Simmons and Nancy Garwood deserve special thanks for their secretarial and organizational help with the volume. Finally, we thank the contributors to this volume; their chapters, critiques, flexibility, and collegiality made this book possible and our collaboration enjoyable.

T. G. Burish
S. M. Levy
B. E. Meyerowitz

1 Cancer, Nutrition, and Eating Behavior: Introduction and Overview

Beth E. Meyerowitz
Thomas G. Burish
Vanderbilt University

Sandra M. Levy
University of Pittsburgh School of Medicine

Cancer causes 20% of all deaths in this country, making the disease the second leading cause of death. The American Cancer Society (1983) estimated that in 1983 855,000 new cases of cancer were identified in the United States. Over half of the people who develop cancer are expected to die within five years from the time of their diagnosis. Moreover, even those people who eventually recover from cancer face major life disruptions as a result of the disease and its treatments. In short, millions of Americans are affected by cancer, its treatment, and its aftermath.

Nutritional status plays a major role in the morbidity and mortality associated with cancer. A leading cause of death in cancer patients is cachexia, a syndrome characterized by malnutrition and progressive physical wasting (Lindsey, Piper, & Stotts, 1982). Not only does malnutrition lead directly to death, but it can also jeopardize indirectly the well-being of patients by causing reductions in the doses of potentially life-saving therapy that patients can tolerate. Malnutrition can also compromise host stamina in other ways; for example, by affecting immunological function, rendering the individual susceptible to infections. In addition, nutrition may play a role in the onset of cancer. A growing number of foods have been identified as contributing to the development of cancer. Thus, cancer can be both a cause and an effect of poor nutrition.

The role of nutrition in the prevention and treatment of cancer has begun only recently to receive empirical and theoretical attention. In 1982 the National Cancer Advisory Board Ad Hoc Subcommittee on Nutrition and Cancer (NCAB, 1982) concluded that insufficent emphasis had been placed on research in diet, nutrition, and cancer. Their report stated that "*Research in nutrition and cancer is at an evolutionary stage in its development.* It needs to bring new sciences and scientists into the field and persuade them to apply their technologies to cancer research. It has to conceive and implement multidisciplinary research approaches. . . ." (p. 13, emphasis in original).

In this volume we provide such a multidisciplinary approach to one determinant of nutritional status–eating behavior. Individuals' abilities to eat and the foods that they choose to consume contribute to health status both before and after the diagnosis of cancer. Understanding, measuring, and modifying eating behavior have been goals of psychological research for decades. In this book, basic biobehavioral research on the role of learning in determining eating behavior is reviewed and its implications for understanding the relation between nutrition and cancer are explored. Before providing an overview of the volume, we briefly discuss factors that affect the nutritional status of cancer patients and the role of nutrition in cancer etiology.

NUTRITIONAL STATUS OF CANCER PATIENTS

Malnutrition is the most common secondary diagnosis in cancer patients (Harvey, Bothe, & Blackburn, 1979). More than one-half of all cancer patients experience cancer cachexia or physical wasting and the nutritional deficits associated with it (Lindsey, Piper, & Stotts, 1982). Cachexia may be the most prevalent immediate cause of death among cancer patients (Theologides, 1977), and improved nutrition may be associated with decreased mortality rates (Harvey et al., 1979).

Nutritional status among cancer patients is influenced by the tumor itself and by various treatments and their side effects (e.g., Chencharick & Mossman, 1983; Donaldson & Lenon, 1979). In general, cachexia is the result of a negative energy balance in which food intake is not adequate to meet the metabolic needs of the host. This condition can be caused by increased energy utilization, decreased food intake, or both (Theologides, 1979). In the case of many cancer patients, both mechanisms play critical roles.

Cancer-caused increases in energy requirements and changes in carbohydrate, protein, and lipid metabolism are well documented. However, these changes do not account entirely for weight loss. As Bernstein (1982) has pointed out, under most circumstances organisms compensate for increased or inefficient energy expenditure by increasing their food intake. Cancer patients rarely increase food intake and, in fact, are more likely to reduce the amount of food they eat.

Although the specific causes of diminished food intake in tumor-bearing organisms are not completely understood, a number of explanations have been offered. Occasionally, observed disruptions in eating behavior can be attributed to obstructions or other mechanical problems in the head and neck region or in the gastrointestinal tract (Lindsey, Piper, & Stotts, 1982). Most disruption in eating, however, probably results from problems that are more closely tied to psychobiologic mechanisms. Changes in chemoreceptors that lead to alterations in taste and smell, and accumulation of food in the intestinal tract that causes a feeling of fullness have been identified as possible determinants of reduced food intake (DeWys, 1979).

Eating behavior is also affected by the side effects of cancer treatments. For example, radiation to the head and neck area can alter taste acuity, produce mouth sores, and make swallowing difficult; and treatment with chemotherapy can produce a variety of gastrointestinal problems including diarrhea, nausea, and vomiting. In addition, the emotional distress, depression, and fatigue that many patients experience when diagnosed or treated for cancer may also lead to anorexia or loss of desire to eat (Neumann, Jelliffe, Zerfas, & Jelliffe, 1982). Finally, changes in eating patterns can result from learned taste aversions (Bernstein, 1982), a process whereby gastric illness can lead to the avoidance of foods that were ingested prior to the illness. These and other possible determinants of decreased food intake in cancer patients are a major focus of this volume.

Although cancer and its treatment often result in decreased food intake, increased nutritional ingestion may not automatically improve the patient's resistance to the cancer or increase his or her ability to withstand more aggressive anticancer treatments. On the contrary, improved nutrition may feed the tumor more than the host, and thus may increase the proliferation rate of the cancer cells (see Levine, this volume).

NUTRITION AND CANCER ETIOLOGY

Nutritional status is not only influenced by cancer and its treatments, it can also contribute to cancer's development. In a recent report on diet, nutrition, and cancer by the National Research Council (described in Maugh, 1982), it was estimated that approximately one-third of the cancers in this country could be prevented through dietary modification. The rate may be even higher for cancers specific to women such as breast or endometrial cancers (Marks, 1977). Epidemiologic research and laboratory experimentation with animals have led to the identification of a number of foods that appear to be associated with an increased or decreased risk for specific cancers. For example, dietary fat, smoked and salt-cured foods, mold contaminated foods (such as nuts and cheese), and burned foods have been linked to cancer (Ames, 1983; Maugh, 1982). Natural mutagens and carcinogens have also been identified in a variety of commonly ingested vegetables and herbs (Ames, 1983). In contrast, other vegetables, specifically those in the Cruciferae family (such as broccoli and cabbage), as well as foods containing β-carotene, selenium, and Vitamins C or E appear to have anticarcinogenic properties (Ames, 1983). Clearly, clinical trials that test directly the causal relationship between these foods and the incidence of cancer in humans are critically important. These studies can also demonstrate the feasibility of enlisting compliance from large numbers of people in changing dietary habits.

ORGANIZATION OF THIS VOLUME

This volume is divided into three sections that explore the role of nutrition and eating behavior in cancer: (1) basic processes in taste aversions and eating behavior; (2) taste aversions and eating behavior in cancer; and (3) interventions for improving the nutritional status of cancer patients and for modifying the diet of populations at high risk for developing cancer.

In the first section, basic biobehavioral research into selective processes underlying eating behavior is reviewed. Robertson and Garcia review the animal research on learned taste aversions. They explain why, for example, animals that ingest certain foods or beverages and then receive X–ray radiation will subsequently develop an aversion to those foods or beverages. The authors then discuss how this basic learning process may occur in cancer patients who receive radiation or chemotherapy. Their chapter highlights the role that learning can play in altering the eating behavior of organisms who are exposed to aversive radiation or chemical substances, and thus how psychological or behavioral factors can interact with biological processes to disrupt eating patterns. In the next chapter, Grunberg argues that learned taste aversions provide only a partial explanation for the altered eating behavior patterns shown by cancer patients. He suggests that many eating problems result from altered taste preferences. Specifically, he presents data from research with both animals and humans which demonstrate that nicotine can alter taste preferences in noncancer-bearing organisms. The author then discusses how cancer may also produce changes in taste preferences and how these changes may lead to decreased caloric intake and weight loss. Grunberg concludes by suggesting methods for overcoming the negative effects of altered taste preferences and for reversing the weight loss that such alterations may cause.

While the first section focuses primarily on basic biobehavioral processes underlying eating disorders in cancer-free animal and human populations, the focus of the second section is on nutritional and eating problems specifically associated with cancer. Research is reviewed that applies the basic mechanisms described in the first section to cancer patients. Bernstein and Treneer, for example, demonstrate that tumor growth per se can result in learned aversions to food. The authors speculate about the physiological basis for this phenomenon, suggesting that certain amino acid deficiencies caused by some tumors can lead to the development of learned food aversions and can result in substantial weight loss. On the basis of their hypotheses, the authors suggest straightforward dietary supplementation procedures that they believe can be effective in preventing and alleviating weight loss among cancer patients. In the next chapter, Smith, Blumsack, and Bilek discuss the role of radiation therapy in the development of taste aversions. They describe a series of studies in which the traditional research paradigm for studying radiation as a cause of learned taste aversions in rats was modified to approximate the experience of cancer radiotherapy patients. These studies demonstrate that under radiotherapy-like conditions, rats learn long-lasting aversions to both unfamiliar and familiar tastes. When conditioned aversions are studied in patients receiving radiation therapy, conditioning also appears to have some effect on eating behavior. The authors discuss possible mechanisms underlying changes in eating behavior and offer recommendations for the prevention of learned taste aversions in radiotherapy patients. In the next chapter, Bernstein and Webster demonstrate that anorexia and altered food preferences can be learned effects of gastrointestinally toxic cancer chemotherapy. They present clinical data from adult and child chemotherapy patients and laboratory data from animals that document the occurrence of learned taste aversions to unfamiliar and familiar foods. Research that explores possible intervention strategies for preventing the development of aversions is also described. In the final chapter of this section, Redd, Burish, and Andrykowski explain how conditioning can cause some chemotherapy patients to experience nausea and vomiting even before their chemotherapy medication is administered, and other patients to display postchemotherapy nausea and vomiting that are more severe than their disease state and treatment protocol would typically induce. These conditioned side effects are experienced by over 25% of cancer chemotherapy patients and can severely compromise the eating behavior and nutritional status of these patients. Included in the chapter is a review of the literature on prevalence rates, underlying mechanisms, and individual differences in the development of conditioned nausea and vomiting.

The third section of the volume focuses on intervention strategies for optimizing the nutritional status of people with cancer or for altering dietary intake of individuals at high risk for developing the disease. DeWys begins the section with an overview of cachexia in cancer patients. He points out that 30% to 90% of cancer patients, depending on tumor type, experience weight loss. Moreover, weight loss is a major prognostic factor, associated with shorter survival and inadequate response to treatment. Clearly, the high incidence and serious consequences of weight loss make effective preventive strategies critically important. DeWys' description of the extent and nature of the problem and of its pathophysiology provide a useful context for understanding intervention strategies. In the next chapter, Bright-See and Levy discuss methodological issues that require consideration when measuring eating behavior and designing interventions to change such behavior. They describe strategies that are appropriate with healthy individuals and with patients with early stage cancers, including strategies for large scale dietary intervention trials with high risk populations. They also discuss techniques for measuring the intake of various foods and food components that are thought to be either carcinogenic or anticarcinogenic. The chapter ends with a brief discussion of issues that are relevant to teaching clinical and research skills in the area of nutrition and cancer.

Following the introduction and perspective provided by DeWys and by Bright-See and Levy, there are three chapters which present specific intervention strategies for influencing nutritional status in relation to cancer. First, Boyd, Cousins, Bayliss, Fish, Fishnell, and Bruce describe an ongoing dietary modification program for cancer prevention. They outline procedures by which they were able to design and implement a program that was successful in markedly reducing the level of dietary fat consumed by women at high risk for breast cancer. Epidemiologic and animal research suggest that this reduction will minimize risk for breast cancer, an hypothesis that Boyd and his colleagues will test. In the next chapter Levine describes a strategy for circumventing the need to change eating behavior in chemotherapy patients. He reviews the literature and presents two studies that test the effects of total parenteral nutrition (TPN), a treatment that provides necessary nutrients to patients intravenously. These studies suggest that although TPN leads to weight gain, it does not appear to increase significantly the survival of chemotherapy patients. Levine also identifies the methodological limitations of these studies and suggests improvements for future research. Finally, Burish, Redd, and Carey provide a critical review of the literature on treatments that have been used to minimize the conditioned nausea, vomiting and emotional distress associated with cancer chemotherapy. They also recommend several strategies for making behavioral interventions more effective and efficient.

SUMMARY AND CONCLUSIONS

Problems such as anorexia, cachexia, learned food aversions, and conditioned nausea and vomiting are frequent and substantial clinical disorders that exert a major impact, directly and indirectly, on cancer morbidity and mortality. Moreover, certain eating habits can promote or interfere with the development of cancer. These nutritional problems and eating behaviors are observable, measurable phenomena that are best understood from an interdisciplinary perspective that integrates both basic and applied research. The present volume was developed with this perspective in mind. It moves from a consideration of basic biobehavioral research on factors that disrupt normal eating behavior to a consideration of specific eating and nutritional problems associated with the development and progression of cancer. By applying basic biobehavioral principles to clinical problems involving cancer and nutrition, a greater understanding of these clinical problems can be gained and new and effective treatment approaches can be developed. This volume does not and could not provide solutions to all of the nutritional problems associated with cancer. However, it does suggest some solutions, and we hope that it also raises questions that will stimulate the additional research that is needed to develop and test other solutions to these critically important problems.

ACKNOWLEDGMENT

The authors thank Shelly Chaiken for her helpful comments on an earlier draft of the chapter. The writing of this chapter was supported in part by Grant No. 25516 from the National Cancer Institute.

REFERENCES

American Cancer Society (1983). *Cancer facts and figures.* New York: American Cancer Society.

Ames, B. N. (1983). Dietary carcinogens and anticarcinogens. *Science, 221,* 1256–1264.

Bernstein, I. L. (1982). Physiological and psychological mechanisms of cancer anorexia. *Cancer Research, 42,* 715s–720s.

Chencharick, J. D., & Mossman, K. L. (1983). Nutritional consequences of the radiotherapy of head and neck cancer. *Cancer, 51,* 811–815.

DeWys, W. D. (1979). Anorexia as a general effect of cancer. *Cancer, 43,* 2013–2019.

Donaldson, S. S., & Lenon, R. A. (1979). Alterations of nutritional status: Impact of chemotherapy and radiation treatment. *Cancer, 43,* 2036–2052.

Harvey, K. B., Bothe, A., Jr., & Blackburn, G. L. (1979). Nutritional assessment and patient outcome during oncological therapy. *Cancer, 43,* 2065–2069.

Lindsey, A. M., Piper, B. F., & Stotts, N. A. (1982). The phenomenon of cancer cachexia: A review. *Oncology Nursing Forum, 9,* 38–42.

Marks, D. A. (1977). Nutrition and the cancer problem: An overview. In M. Winick (Ed.), *Current concepts in nutrition: Vol. 6. Nutrition and cancer* (pp. 7–13). New York: Wiley.

Maugh, T. H. (1982). Cancer is not inevitable. *Science, 217,* 36–37.

National Cancer Advisory Board (1982). *Report of the National Cancer Advisory Board Ad Hoc Subcommittee on Nutrition and Cancer.* Bethesda, MD: National Cancer Institute.

Neumann, C. G., Jelliffe, D. B., Zerfas, A. J., & Jelliffe, E. F. P. (1982). Nutritional assessment of the child with cancer. *Cancer Research, 42,* 699s–712s.

Theologides, A. Cancer cachexia. In M. Winick (Ed.), *Current Concepts in nutrition: Vol. 6 Nutrition and Cancer* (pp. 75–94). New York: Wiley.

Theologides, A. (1979). Cancer cachexia. *Cancer, 43,* 2004–2012.

I

BASIC PROCESSES IN TASTE AVERSIONS AND EATING BEHAVIOR

2 X–Rays and Learned Taste Aversions: Historical and Psychological Ramifications

Rodrigo Garcia y Robertson
Villanova University

John Garcia
University of California at Los Angeles

INTRODUCTION AND OVERVIEW

This chapter presents an historical discussion of the impact of medical X–rays on psychology, with an emphasis on implications for understanding the changed eating behavior and emesis often observed in cancer patients. Despite early convictions to the contrary, X–rays proved to be both perceptible and injurious. The discovery of these qualities suggested that X–rays might affect organisms psychologically, and led to an interest in the impact of X–rays on learning. A considerable body of research has demonstrated that animals do, indeed, demonstrate new learning as a result of undergoing radiation. Their learning, however, cannot be understood by reference to traditional, strictly associationistic learning principles. As we demonstrate, it is only by viewing learning within an evolutionary context that the findings from the X–ray experiments can be explained.

Perhaps the most striking findings regarding learning and X–rays involve the learning that results from the gastrointestinal distress caused by X–rays. In the second half of this chapter we focus on the application of a new, adaptive view of learning generated by the X–ray research to the psychobiology of emesis and learned taste aversions. Since gastrointestinal distress is a common result of many cancer therapies, these findings can have important implications for cancer patients. We conclude with a discussion of these implications.

In order to present a comprehensive picture of the impact of X–rays we integrate several perspectives. Because nearly a century has passed since the invention of the X–ray tube, which emitted a new unknown stimulus, this chapter provides an historical review. The scientist's perception of a new phenomena is colored by preconceptions and motivations, so this chapter will be in part a sociological discussion. And, because no phenomenon or concept is completely without precedent, we delve into the history of psychology to find the skeins of psychological thought which lead to a theoretical reformulation capable of accounting for the new empirical facts uncovered in the wake of the X–stimulus.

History has imposed a certain social structure upon medical research with ionizing radiation. Research began within the purview of physics, but with the advent of the X–ray discharge tube medical scientists and practitioners took over. Basic research on animals conducted by biologists first met with some rebuffs, but their contributions were soon considered essential. Psychologists were the last to enter radiation research and, as often happens with newcomers, they entered at the bottom of hierarchial interdisciplinary research teams and had to establish the legitimacy of their scientific inquiries. As a result, the X–stimulus and subsequent radiation and cancer research are only now making a theoretical impact upon psychology.

ON THE STRUCTURE OF S–R LEARNING THEORY

In order to appreciate the theoretical and practical problems created for psychology by the X–ray data, one must keep in mind the rigid associationistic structure of traditional learning theory. By 1950, learning or conditioning theory had developed a series of abstract laws which presumably applied to any stimulus (S) evoking any response (R) in any organism (O). These S–R laws, carefully constructed on a huge experimental data base, were essentially parametric definitions of the three principles of association formalized by the empirical philosophers of the sixteenth and seventeenth century. As applied to any two elements (S–S, S–R, R–S, R–R) they were: (1) the association by similarity of the two elements; (2) the association by cause and effect relationships between the two elements; and (3) the association by contiguity of the two elements in time and space. Experimental psychologists were so successful at controlling the behavior of animals utilizing these principles that the principles were elevated to the status of universal "laws" of learning.

The Law of Similarity has played a relatively minor role in learning theory. Similarity forms the basis for generalization from one learning element to another, or conversely, for discrimination between one element and another. Although the data generated by X–ray research has presented some problems for this law, there has been at least one inadequate attempt to absorb the new information from the radiation laboratories, and some chemotherapy clinics, by appealing to the Law of Similarity, (Testa, 1974).

Association by cause and effect was reformulated by modern experimenters as the "Law of Effect." In the classical (S–S) association model, the first S is a signal which catches the attention of the organism. It is called the conditioned stimulus (CS). The second S, called the unconditioned stimulus (US), is a stimulus which reliably goads the organism into a reflexive action called the unconditioned response (UR). After conditional pairing of the CS and US, the CS elicits a newly acquired reaction called the conditioned response (CR). The CR is functionally related to the UR and, in essence, it is an anticipatory adaptation to the US evoked by the CS after learning. In the instrumental conditioning model (R–S), the CR is viewed as a habit formed association of any R emitted by O which is followed by a reinforcing S. Reinforcement is produced by a "satisfying" state of affairs such as in obtaining a reward or terminating a punishment. This is the context in which accommodation must be made for the effect of the X–stimulus on a mammalian organism. As we will see, this association will require discarding the traditional views of the S, R, and O, and formulation of new psychological concepts based on the evolutional nature of the specific organism under study.

Association by contiguity of S–S, S–R, or R–R was an extremely important law, and it was here that the X–stimulus made its most crushing impact. As formulated by modern experimental psychologists, contiguity means that if an association between two elements is to be learned, the two elements must be contiguous, that is, separated in time by no more than seconds, or separated in space by no more than "centimeters." Experimenters amassed a great deal of evidence using arbitrary CSs and USs demonstrating that contiguity within this narrow temporal or spatial range is a *sufficient* condition for associative learning under a wide range of conditions. But radiation research has demonstrated that contiguity is not a *necessary* condition for learning, thereby restricting the generality of the contiguity principle, and requiring theorists to specify boundary conditions for this grand old law.

In summary, psychological reactions to X–ray exposure proved to be a kind of conditioning or learning that did not conform well to any of the three "laws" of association. As a result, radiation research, which began as an "applied area," moved to center stage as "basic research" in psychological theory. The specific purposes of the present chapter are fourfold: (1) To comment on the first conflicting opinions on the X–ray invention which set the precedent for later conflicts; (2) to describe in some detail the experiments that defined the properties of the new X–stimulus that were crucial to psychology; (3) to discuss the physiological side-effects of cancer treatment upon the feeding system and nutrition, and (4) to present a reformulation of psychological learning theory encompassing these new data.

TWO HISTORIC X–RAY CONTROVERSIES

In 1895, Wilhelm Conrad Roentgen described an apparatus which yielded "a new kind of ray," thereby welding physics and biology into a new applied area, Health Physics, and creating a new medical specialization, Radiology. This apparatus was apparently the fulfillment of an age-old medical and scientific desire to visualize internal organs of the living body in a nonevasive way. The most wishful beliefs were that new "X–light" would: (1) pass through sensory organs without stimulating them; and (2) illuminate the internal organs without damaging them. Almost immediately there was evidence that X–rays could cause damage, but the evidence was discounted or simply ignored, and then rediscovered again and again as the new technology moved from physics to physiology and ultimately to psychology. Setting an example for those who followed, Roentgen exposed his own flesh to the "new rays" and described the effect as follows: "If one hand be held between the discharge-tube and the screen, the darker shadow of the bones is seen within the slightly dark shadow-image of the hand itself" (Baker, 1899, pp. 3–4).

The shadow cast by Roentgen's hand portended a host of biological applications for the new X–ray machines, and the enthusiasm generated by Roentgen's words set off a scramble to probe every facet of living tissue with the new rays. Hands were quickly followed by limbs, lungs, stomachs, and brains. Early investigators varied from a fifteen-year-old boy, Francis Le Roy Satterlee, who X–rayed his father's hand eleven days after Roentgen's formal presentation of his first X–ray paper, to Benjamin Franklin Thomas, Chair of Physics at Ohio State, who submitted to hours of X–rays in order to map the lower thoracic and upper lumbar vertebrae (Brown, 1936).

On Visual Perception of X-rays

The most popular belief, at least before the dawn of the atomic age, was that X–ray was not a stimulus. It was considered colorless, odorless, and tasteless. Today we know that this notion is probably wrong on all counts. The controversy concerning sensory effects began with vision. In his first communication on the X–ray apparatus Roentgen commented that: "The retina of the eye is not sensitive to the rays. Even if the eye is close to the discharge tube, it observes nothing, although, as experiment has proved, the media contained in the eye must be sufficiently transparent to transmit the rays" (Baker, 1899, p. 7).

When another pioneer of X–ray research reported visual responses to the X–ray beam without the aid of the fluorescent paper screen, Roentgen recalled his own faint visual sensations which he had dismissed as subjective illusions (Baker, 1899). Using X–ray tubes which yielded more intense rays, he tested his own eye again. In his second paper, he reported on his own intriguing perceptual experiment:

> If a vertical metal slit some tenths of a millimeter broad is held as close as possible before the open or closed eye, and if the head, completely enveloped in a black cloth, is then brought near the discharge apparatus, there is observed, after some practice, a weak, nonuniformly bright strip of light which, according to the place

> where the slit is in front of the eye, takes a different form—straight, curved or circular. By a slow motion of the slit in a horizontal direction, these different forms can be made to pass gradually from one to the other. An explanation of the phenomena is found immediately if we consider that the ball of the eye is cut by a lamellar sheaf of X–rays. (Baker, 1899, pp. 39–40)

Even Roentgen's reputation was not enough to permanently establish the visability of X–rays in the minds of the scientific community. In fact, the opposite notion, that X–rays and other forms of ionizing radiation were first and foremost invisible, became well established in the literature. William Rollins, whose privately published *Notes on X–light* is an invaluable early compilation of X–ray data, stated quite routinely that X–rays were an "invisible radiation of which none of our senses make us conscious" (Rollins, 1903). S. P. Thompson (1921) classed X–rays as invisible light in *Light Visible and Invisible.* Some investigators disagreed, such as A. H. Compton (1935) who described a "faint effect upon the retina." But the more common view was that expressed by H. M. Muncheryan (1940), that the primary property of X–rays was that they were invisible.

However, according to L. E. Lipetz (1955), Axenfeld reported in 1896 that insects and crustaceans in a dark chamber moved towards radiation soon after the onset of exposure. Blinded invertebrates did not, so the clear implication was that ionizing rays produced a visual sensation in these phototropic subjects. More recent studies established the case beyond doubt. Newell and Borley (1941) used an elegant technique, reminescent of Roentgen's second report, to ascertain the visual acuity of patients with cataractous eyes. Eventually, Kimeldorf and Hunt (1965) were able to review a mass of evidence on visual effects of ionizing rays. Finally, in a fascinating experiment, D'Arcy and Porter (1962) demonstrated that human observers, trained by operant conditioning methods, could respond to cosmic particles detected by a Geiger tube. The subjects described the "cosmic hit" as a bright point of light. Nevertheless, when astronauts reported sparks and streaks during lunar exploration voyages, NASA officials were puzzled. On later Apollo flights, the light flashes were verified by the dark-adapted and blindfolded observers and the visual effects were tentatively attributed to cosmic ray nuclei penetrating the head and eyes of the astronauts (Pinsky, Osborne, Bailey, Benson, & Thompson, 1974). We now know that tiny X–ray doses of less than one roentgen (r) can produce the greenish glow seen by humans. Nor are we alone in this; monkeys view X–rays in much the same way (Chaddock, 1972).

On Injury From X–ray Exposure

The second X–ray controversy involved reluctance to attribute biological damage to X–ray exposure. Evolution had probably not prepared the human mind to perceive danger in an intangible glow emanating from a distant source not in contact with the body. But within 90 days of Roentgen's announcement of the discovery of X–rays, examples of radiological damage were appearing in the literature. These, in turn, were quickly attacked in a number of ways. The editors of *Nature* quoted the experiences of A. C. C. Smith and J. C. M. Stanton as testimony against optical damage by X–rays (Brown, 1936). Telsa wrote in the *Electrical Review,* that the burns attributed to X–rays were really due to ozone and nitric acid (Rollins, 1903). M. K. Kassabian attacked the use of the word "burn" to describe the injuries, for fear that the word might have the wrong connotations (Brown, 1936). Others contended that sores and scars on the hands were caused not by the radiation, but by the chemicals used to develop X–ray plates.

Researchers clashed with clinicians. Rollins (1903) reported that guinea pigs subjected to prolonged radiation exposure died, while unexposed controls continued to thrive. Codman (1901), a surgeon at Massachusetts General Hospital in charge of X–ray at the Children's Hospital, dismissed the experimental evidence commenting, "The fact that the X–ray is in daily use in the large hospitals without harmful results should be put in blacker type than the death of two guinea pigs." Rollins (1903) dismissed the clinical evidence, commenting that "An experiment can only be discredited by another experiment."

The pioneers in medical X–ray unflinchingly paid a grim price for their courageous exploration of this valuable diagnostic tool. Codman (1901) was suffering from the first stages of X–ray burns when he noted, "One severe case of maiming dermatitis I have seen, in a gentleman whose enthusiasm outweighed his prudence, but the value of whose work has almost compensated for this sacrifice." He was probably referring to his colleague at Massachusetts General Hospital, W. J. Dodd, who continued his X–ray work despite crippling pains in his hands. Dodd and some other early practitioners apparently died for their belief that the patient's benefits outweighed the risk to the physician. For example, Kassabian's fatal carcinoma began in the same left hand that he habitually placed under the X–ray to calm the fears of his patients. And Thomas, who exposed himself to hours of X–rays in order to minimize patient complaints, also died from carcinoma (Brown, 1936).

Here, there appears to be a gap of several decades in our story because the emphasis on research turned away from the stimulus property of ionizing radiation. The capacity of ionizing radiation to injure living tissue became the focus of research in physiology and medicine. That capacity to produce relatively permanent injury became a useful tool for research and treatment when it was demonstrated that proliferating and migrating cells were more susceptible to radiation damage than mature stable cells. By exposing developing mammalian embryos to ionizing rays at different stages of development, individuals with specific brain deformities could be produced and tested for physiological and behavioral integrity (Altman, 1975; Rugh, 1962). In the same general way, neoplastic tissue is more susceptible than normal tissue, thus X–rays became a standard treatment for rapidly growing tumors. Chemical agents having similar (radiomimetic) effects on proliferating tumors were developed as alternative treatment strategies. This work was of immense scientific and medical importance, but this chapter deals with the relatively immediate effects of radiation exposure (or of injections of radiomimetic drugs and emetic toxins) which directly promote a unique form of conditioning or learning.

THE X-STIMULUS STUDIED PSYCHOLOGICALLY

The Questions Posed by Psychologists

The psychological research program at the U.S. Naval Radiological Defense Laboratory on Hunter's Point in San Francisco Bay began around 1950 under the direction of D. J. Kimeldorf, a physiological radiobiologist, and E. L. Hunt, an experimental psychologist. The laboratory was a converted building which retained the ambiance of its former existence as U.S. Navy Jail or "brig." Attitudes towards radiation damage had changed with the beginning of the "atomic age," replete with cyclotrons, atomic bombs, lasers and potential "death rays." X–rays caused "radiation sickness" and accelerated particles left tracks of damage as they coursed through animal tissue. The question which haunted physicist and physician alike was put to the psychologist: "Will exposure of brain and tissue to ionizing rays produce psychological changes in animals and people? Will exposure derange memory and change personality?"

Many comparisons were made between the performance of irradiated animals and nonirradiated animals, but little progress was made until experimental psychologists recast the older, more fundamental questions within their own S–R methodology. So phrased, these two questions were: (1) Can radiation serve as a US to establish learned habits in animals? (2) Can radiation be used as a CS to signal an animal? Though these questions may seem innocuous, their implica-. tions raised the ire of some scientists with much radiation experience and knowledge. Observing no arousal or avoidance in their animal subjects, they questioned the usefulness of psychological questions and rejected the very notion that their animals could learn about radiation. Other radiological scientists pointed out that these empirical tests had not been carried out appropriately, therefore psychological experiments might reveal new knowledge.

Experiments Using X–rays as a Toxic US

The research in the brig actually began with gamma rays which, for our purposes, are the same as X–rays from a high energy source. The rays emanated from a brass capsule containing about seven curies of cobalt 60. The capsule was attached to the tip of a rod and rested in the center of a lead ball during the "off" condition. During the "on" condition the capsule was withdrawn from the lead sphere and rotated by an electric motor to ensure a uniform exposure field. The research mission was to determine the effects of long exposures at low intensities as might be encountered by a population in an area of radioactive debris from an atomic explosion.

To isolate the *stimulus* properties of the gamma rays, a host of new procedures were set in motion. Rats had to be alert and comfortable during exposure, so each rat was confined to an individual plastic box with a water spout and food pellets available during the eight hours of exposure. Radiation dose decreases as the distance from the cobalt 60 increases, so experimental animals were placed in boxes at fixed distances to control the dose. Control animals were confined to similar boxes in the "shadow" of a stack of lead bricks and subjected to all the other stimuli associated with exposure except for the major portion of the direct hits of the gamma rays emanating from the source. The walls of the brig and the mechanical structures within the room produced a high background radiation level even in the shadow of the lead brick wall due to scattering and diffusion of the gamma rays. The rays also interacted with the air producing ozone and similar odorants which circulated behind the bricks. In addition, the controls were exposed to the same machinery noises which could disturb the animals' feeding behavior. Needless to say, many other scientists were not always favorably impressed with our obsessive concerns for the rats' psyches.

In the first studies, we simply recorded the amount of food and water consumed and the body weight change for each animal during the 8-hour exposure to gamma rays.[1] The rate of exposure was 9.4r per hour and the total dose was 75 r per exposure. This radiation treatment was repeated once a week for eight weeks. Water consumption showed a steady decline with each exposure, so that by the seventh and eighth exposures the experimental animals were virtually not drinking during confinement. Food consumption was depressed, but the progressive decline was not so dramatic; it seemed that the animals were refusing water, leading to a reduction in their dry food intake, and a loss in body weight. It appeared that the radiation made the animals ill, causing a decrease in their normal water and food consumption. After a series of exposures, the animals inexplicably reduced their consumption whenever they were confined in the brig, *even in the absence of radiation*. Obviously, the rats had been conditioned by the gamma rays, but how?

At this juncture, serendipity played its hand. In the home cage, rats drank from glass bottles, but during radiation they drank from plastic test tubes which could be attached more conveniently to the small boxes in which they were confined during exposure. This seemingly trivial variable did more to reveal the

[1] "We" usually refers to an interdisciplinary research team composed of various individuals on which the Psychobiologist (John Garcia) was the Principal Investigator and the Historian (Rodrigo Garcia y Robertson) served as a young volunteer on occasion.

psychological nature of radiation exposure than all our ratiocinative maneuvers. Acting on a sudden impulse, we took the glass water bottle off a rat's home cage as it was drinking avidly and offered it a drink from the plastic test tube. The effects were dramatic. Upon tasting the water, the thirsty animal jerked its head back, groomed its muzzle vigorously, rubbed its chin on the floor of its cage and refused to drink again. When we offered it the glass bottle, it sampled the water and then licked vigorously again; when we switched back to the plastic test tube the animal again refused to drink in obvious frustration.

We were certain that the rat was reacting to a taste imparted to the water by the plastic test tube. Since the plastic test tube was used during radiation exposure, we hypothesized that the taste of the water became associated with the illness induced by radiation and as a result of this association it also became aversive and animals avoided it. Our colleagues pointed out that we had no independent evidence that water had a "plastic taste" or even that the rats were ill during exposure; most reports from human patients indicated that radiation illness, if it occurred, came hours after exposure, much too late to produce a learned aversion. Current S–R wisdom dictated that the taste CS would have to be followed immediately by the noxious US if an association between them was to be formed according to the "Law of Contiguity."

We designed an experiment to test the taste aversion hypothesis using a known taste as a CS thus eliminating the "plastic taste" presumption. We placed plastic tubes on all our rats' home cages as well as on the radiation box, so that the plastic was a constant factor and no longer uniquely paired with radiation exposure. As the taste CS, we selected a solution of one gram of saccharin powder to one liter of water. This very sweet fluid was highly preferred by rats; reversing a strong preference would be convincing evidence that exposure to ionizing rays produced a conditioned aversion.

For our first saccharin study we divided the rats into six groups. Each group was tested for saccharin preference. Saccharin was quite popular; given a free choice, most of the rats chose saccharin-flavored water for over 85% of their fluid intake. The six groups were then divided into three pairs; in each paired group, one received saccharin-flavored water during exposure and the other group received tap water. To eliminate any chance that the animals were responding to any stimulus other than the radiation, they all went through the same testing routine with only the radiation dose differing for each pair of groups. One pair of groups received a 57r dose of gamma rays over 6 hours of exposure, the next pair 30r and the final pair zero r. The results were instructive. Both zero dose groups retained their high preference for saccharin. So did those rats that were irradiated but drank tap water during exposure. Results were dramatically different for those rats that drank saccharin during exposure. Those rats whose saccharin intake was coupled with 30r of gamma rays dropped their saccharin intake by around 70% in the posttest and those exposed to 57r while drinking saccharin cut their intake by over 90%. Furthermore, the saccharin aversions endured for over a month of testing during which the animals had both tap water and saccharine water continuously available in their home cages (Garcia, Kimeldorf, & Koelling, 1955).

Summary of the US Effects

This experiment initiated a large number of studies in which ionizing rays and accelerated particles served as USs in psychological experiments. The original results were replicated and extended. (For early reviews, see Garcia, Kimeldorf, & Hunt, 1961; Kimeldorf & Hunt, 1965.) Smith, Blumsak, & Bilek (this volume) provide us with a more recent review of this literature—a literature to which they have made many significant contributions. We will here only summarize the principal characteristics of X–ray as a US and its underlying neurophysiological mechanisms.

1. X–rays produce a selective effect. Animals acquire strong aversions for tastes associated with exposure, but they do not fear the radiation compartment. However, rats display a mild preference for the nonirradiated compartment when given a choice (Garcia, Kimeldorf, & Hunt, 1957).
2. The taste aversion is a function of the total dose accumulated rather than the intensity of the stimulus, i.e., the dose rate (a total dose of 20r produces about the same effect whether it is delivered in four hours or four minutes). This contrasts sharply with vision for example, where perceived brightness is a function of stimulus intensity (Garcia, Kimeldorf, & Hunt, 1961).
3. The abdomen is the most sensitive area. A collimated beam aimed at the abdomen produces a stronger taste aversion than when directed at any other part of the body (Garcia & Kimeldorf, 1960). Roughly speaking, the same holds true for radiation-induced nausea and emesis in human patients.
4. Blood or serum from irradiated donors will produce taste aversions in recipient rats which drink saccharin prior to transfusion (Garcia, Ervin, & Koelling, 1967; Hunt, Carrol, & Kimeldorf, 1968). This indicates that the US agent is an endogenous product, perhaps histamine, circulating in the blood during and after exposure (Levy, Carrol, Smith, & Hofer, 1974; Levy, Ervin, & Garcia, 1970).
5. Taste aversions can be produced by a variety of agents, other than radiation exposure, which produce nausea. Furthermore, taste aversions can be induced in one trial even when the nauseous treatment is delayed for hours (Garcia, Ervin, & Koelling, 1966; Garcia & Koelling, 1967).

Experiments Using X–rays as an Olfactory CS

Soon another, more immediate, response to X–ray was discovered. Sleeping rats were aroused within 12 seconds of the onset of exposure. Blind rats did the same, eliminating the possibility that visual effects were the arousing stimuli. Hunt and Kimeldorf (1962, 1964) interpreted their results as "evidence for the direct stimulation of the mammalian nervous system." They presented the intriguing hypothesis that X–rays might be acting directly upon synaptic and ganglionic sites throughout the nervous system to arouse the rat from sleep. They came close to postulating a new sensory phenomena. But, the postulation of a "new" sense must pass a rigorous test devised centuries ago as part of "the doctrine of specific energies of the nerves." Johannes Muller is generally credited with the formalization of this doctrine, though he was anticipated in part by John Locke in 1690 (Garcia, 1981) and more completely by Charles Bell in 1811 (Boring, 1950). In a strikingly similar situation, Muller argued that evidence that animals could detect electricity did not indicate an "electrical sense." It merely indicated that the normal senses probably responded to electricity. Muller pointed out: "The essential attribute of a new sense is not the perception of external objects or influences which ordinarily do not act upon the senses, but that external causes should excite in it a new and particular kind of sensation different from all the sensations of the five senses" (Sahakian, 1978, pp. 143–144).

Muller's doctrine is conservative; before postulating a new sense or inventing a nonsequitur such as "extrasensory perception," one must first eliminate the possibility that the transmission of new information occurs via the well-known sensory receptors. Ultimately, rats proved to be sensitive via one of the traditional five senses but the notion of direct stimulation of the central nervous system by the penetrating rays was not disproved, it was merely set aside and forgotten, perhaps to be taken up again at some future date.

In that same year, Garcia, Buchwald, Feder and Koelling (1962) reported on the immediate detection of an X–ray CS by rats trained with Skinnerian techniques and apparati. The Skinner box was a small acoustically-treated compartment equipped with a food delivery apparatus and a response lever. Every 12 lever presses by the rat caused the apparatus to deliver a pellet of food. A cummulative recorder measured response rate, and an electric grid delivered shock to the rat's feet. To mask any extraneous sounds, a speaker flooded the chamber with "white" noise. In addition to the record there was a double pane window to allow visual observation. We placed the entire arrangement under a 250kv X–ray machine, with a 3⁄16 lead plate suspended between it and the box in order to block out radiation between exposures.

Training was a variation of the conditioned suppression procedure (Estes & Skinner, 1941). In preliminary conditioning, the lever was removed and the X–ray CS was paired with electric shock US; about 40 conditioning trials were administered over two or three days. We then installed the food lever for the tests, and testing took place while the rat was actively pressing the lever for food. Swinging away the silent shield exposed the rat to the X–ray CS, but exposure was not followed by the shock US. In many cases, even a brief (10–15 second) exposure immediately suppressed lever pressing. Sham exposures (identical to test exposures except that the copper filter in the X–ray machine was replaced by a lead plate) produced no effect at all. Those rats which did not show conditioned suppression in the first tests were quickly conditioned by a series of discrimination training trials; rats were shocked whenever they pressed the food lever during exposure. Within ten trials all of these animals had learned to suppress lever pressing to the onset of the X–ray CS.

Summary of the CS Effects

These two studies in 1962 demonstrating X–ray arousal and X–ray discrimination in the rat were followed by a series of studies refining the behavioral techniques and adding electrophysiological evidence. The mammalian olfactory mucosa proved to be extremely sensitive to ionizing radiation. This evidence is extensively reviewed by Garcia and Koelling (1971). We will only summarize the unusual properties of this olfactory CS.

1. Animals can immediately detect the onset and offset of the X–ray CS when the beam is directed at the olfactory system. X–ray directed at the nasal air passages anterior to the olfactory receptors is ineffective. On the other hand, intact rats breathing through tracheal tubes respond to X–ray, but olfactory bulbectomies abolish these responses (Garcia, Buchwald, Feder, Koelling, & Tedrow, 1964; Hull, Garcia, Buchwald, Dubrowsky, & Feder, 1965).
2. The magnitude of the X–ray CS is a function of intensity or dose rate. Rats can detect extremely small doses of a few milliroentgens such as might be experienced in dental X–rays (Garcia, Buchwald, Bach-y-Rita, Feder, & Koelling, 1963; Garcia, Buchwald, Hull, & Koelling, 1964).
3. The olfactory receptor can follow a flickering X–ray up to about 10 cycles per second before the flicker fuses into a steady state. Thus, it should be possible to explore the olfactory mucosa with ionizing beams just as the retina has been explored with light beams; regional sensitivity could be assessed and the evoked responses in the brain could be accumulated and averaged as repeated pulses of rays are delivered to selected olfactory targets. For this purpose, weak sources (beta rays) could be used conveniently (Cooper, 1968; Garcia, Green, & McGowan, 1969).

THE X–RAY PARADOX AND LEARNING THEORY

The rats' behavior during exposure to ionizing radiation presented us with the following paradox: X–ray is a potent CS or signal. The onset of exposure stimulates the olfactory receptors arousing sleepy animals. Alert animals orient to the "odor CS" with acute sensitivity. When these brief flashes of X–ray are followed by tiny footshocks, the animals quickly learn to use X–rays as a warning signal in order to avoid the tingle to their feet. Thus they can associate the X–ray CS with an aversive (shock) US.

Despite the fact that rats can perceive the deadly rays they make no great effort to avoid exposure. X–rays are very aversive, producing prompt gastric stasis, delayed abdominal malaise, anemia and ultimately death. In fact, the footshock we used was a trivial annoyance compared to the effect of the rays themselves. Furthermore, a rat can associate a taste CS with a very weak radiation US with astonishing speed and sensitivity. It will acquire an aversion for saccharine-water in a single trial, when that preferred fluid is followed by a long exposure (4 hours) to low intensity radiation (0.0007 r) resulting in a low total dose (10r) (Garcia et al., 1961). Paradoxically, a rat cannot effectively associate the X–ray odor CS with the X–ray aversive US effects although these two stimuli are always paired in the classic CS–US manner during exposure. If repeated brief exposures are not followed by footshock, or anything else of consequence to the rat, the animals habituate within five trials and sleep throughout subsequent exposures (Garcia et al., 1963). Moreover, if a rat is confined in a distinctly bicameral compartment, half exposed and half shielded from radiation, it will, in all probability, accumulate a fatal dose before it learns to stay out of the clearly marked radiation area. It is very poor at associating the tactual, visual and olfactory CSs of the exposed area with a strong radiation US, but it is excellent at associating a taste CS with the same radiation US (Garcia & Koelling, 1967).

There is more to this paradox. The X–ray US has a peculiar latent effect. In one study, five groups of thirsty rats were required to press a lever for saccharine-water during a 30-minute exposure to intensities ranging from trivial to deadly (0.0, 0.005, 0.014, 0.050, 0.450 r/sec). There was no dose effect during exposure; the cumulative response curves were identical for the lowest and the highest intensity groups. However, there was a profound latent effect when the groups were returned to the lever boxes 24 hours later. In the absence of any further exposure, they displayed response decrements varying as a direct function of the dose received the day before (Buchwald, Garcia, Feder, & Bach-y-rita, 1964).

An Adaptive Alternative to S–R Learning Theory

The apparent paradox is a dissonance between the empirical results obtained with X–rays and the rigid abstract associationistic structure of modern learning theory. First, the empirical results demonstrated that there was a powerful *selective* affinity between the X–stimulus and certain classes of other stimuli. For example, rats could readily learn the association between X–ray (US) and taste (CS), but not the association between X–ray and tactual, visual or olfactory stimuli. Prior to this time it was generally held that a US had universal properties such that a US effective with one CS would work with any other CS. The data from the X–ray conditioning studies called this conclusion into question. Second, the powerful law of association by contiguity of the CS–US pairs was somehow circumvented by using the X–stimulus as a US. Prior research had supposedly shown that under a wide range of circumstances, contiguity in time or space is a sufficient condition for associative learning to occur, and specifically with regard to time, contiguity meant seconds or a fraction thereof, not minutes or hours. Yet the X–ray research demonstrated that animals could learn an association between a taste CS and an X–ray (or some other toxic) US even though they were separated in time by hours. Testa (1974) suggested that the X–ray data were not inconsistent with the law of contiguity. He argued that taste-illness conditioning was facilitated because the CS was similar to the US, a taste CS lingering in the oral end of the gastrointestinal tube is more similar to the nauseous effects of the X–ray lingering in the gastric segment of the tube than it is to a place defined by externally referred cues such as sights, sounds, and smells. There is some virtue in this view because it forces one to consider the specific sensory properties of the CS and the US in any given conditioning situation. Ultimately this would lead to an examination of the receptor and the brain terminals at the end of the afferent tracts which transmit the CS and US, which is exactly what we advocate. But as a purely behavioral principle, similarity is not enough. Rapid learning is possible between such dissimilar CS–US pairs as a faint whiff of almond to the nose followed by a sharp pain to the foot, or a tap on the skin followed by the sour taste of vinegar lingering in the mouth.

The rat's behavior in an X–ray field is not paradoxical from an evolutionary perspective which focuses on the structure of organisms. It makes perfect sense. Animals and plants evolved together in a symbiotic complex of coevolution. Animals utilize plants for food and shelter. Plants utilize animals for pollination and dispersal of their fertilized seed. Plants have evolved defenses such as thorns and toxins in their roots, branches and leaves to protect these vital structures from herbivores. The best defense against a hungry herbivore is to turn off its appetite, and by natural selection many plants have evolved bitter emetic toxins which produce that precise effect. In addition, some plants have evolved warning odors and visual signals in conjunction with their bitter toxin. The herbivore evolves compensatory mechanisms by which it learns to avoid a second meal on that particular plant species using odor and visual cues without even taking a bite (Eisner & Grant, 1981). But since plants use animals for their own reproductive purposes, repelling of all herbivores is a poor strategy; differential reinforcement is a better one. Sweet nectar and bright flowers attract insects and birds which inadvertently carry pollen from flower to flower, assisting fertilization. Sweet fruits contain slick indigestible seeds which the herbivore carries in its gut to drop in distant places. Many plants contain both chemical repellants and attractants, so that the discrimination based on taste is an effective evolutionary strategy for any organism in the selection of nutrients and avoidance of toxin.

The natural world in which the rat was selected had few, if any, places which caused illness in the total absence of ingestion and no places where ionizing radiations were powerful enough to cause illness and death. Illness and death might be loosely associated with "places" which are unhealthy for certain species, but even in this case, endogenous conditions usually make mammalian species like the rat vulnerable to external attack. Injury and death come most often from charging predators announced by the sounds of rapid foot falls. Odors reveal the predator in ambush. Movable eyes placed laterally and dorsally on the head perched on a swiveling neck search the sky for avian attacks. A sensitive cutaneous surface is the final defense for most mammals.

The X–ray paradox is thus explained. Due to its heritage, the rat is very effective at relating distal signals with peripheral insults to its skin, therefore it quickly associates the X–ray odor CS with foot-shock. But, a strategy that is very effective for anticipation of danger from one quarter inevitably leaves the organism vulnerable to an unexpected threat from another quarter. The rat is not effective at associating taste to cutaneous insults, or at associating sights and sounds to nausea in the gut. But it is very effective at relating taste of food to poison, and because the X–ray US mimics a poisonous effect, the rat is able to associate a saccharin CS with the X–ray US in a single trial.

On an Experimentus Crusis

The stage was set for a crucial test of two views: From the evolutionary point of view, the rat is a biased learning machine designed by natural selection to form only certain CS-US associations rapidly. From a traditional learning viewpoint, the rat is an unbiased learner able to make any association in accordance with the general principles of contiguity, effect and similarity. A number of experiments were designed and carried out to decide between the two theoretical positions. The results were always in the same direction so we will describe only one which used simple procedures (Garcia, McGowan, Ervin, & Koelling, 1968).

Rats were given food pellets marked either by visual cues or taste cues. For the visual cue, dry food pellets about one inch square were either presented whole as "large" pellets or cut into quarters and presented as "little" pellets. For the taste cue, little pellets were liberally dusted with powdered sugar to make them "sweet," or dusted in flour to look the same but taste "nonsweet." The visual and taste cues were paired with two forms of punishment, either radiation exposure or mild shock to the feet. We tested four independent groups of rats (each group was split into two balanced subgroups):

1. In the visual-shock group, half the animals were punished for eating large pellets with a shock to the feet immediately after lifting the pellet to the mouth; they were allowed to eat the little pellets in safety. Little pellets were paired with shock and large pellets were safe for the other half of the visual-shock group.

2. In the taste-shock group, the same scheme was used. For any given rat, one taste cue was punished and another taste cue was safe, for half the rats sweet was shocked and for the remainder sweet was safe.

3. For the visual-X–ray group, half of the animals were exposed to X–rays (50r) immediately after a meal of big pellets but not after the meals of the little pellets. The remainder was treated conversely with respect to the size cue.

4. For the taste-X–ray group the same balanced scheme was used; for any given rat, one flavor was punished with X–ray and the other was safe.

The animals received a total of five punishment sessions, with one X–ray exposure delivered during each session. Each punishment session was separated by several days of safe sessions to insure a clear discrimination. Several days after the last conditioning session, each rat was tested with its forbidden food. Latency to pick up the first pellet and total amount eaten were recorded.

The visual-shock rats hesitated a long time before picking up the forbidden-size pellet, whereas they had immediately seized the safe pellet on the preceding day. They feared to pick up the pellet, but once having done so they ate it with relish. On the other hand, taste-shock rats learned nothing despite contiguity of the taste CS with the foot-shock US. Taste-X–ray rats learned despite the lack of contiguity between taste and the nauseous effects of X–ray which occurred about an hour or two after exposure. They did not fear to pick up the forbidden-taste pellet, but upon tasting it they rejected it in disgust. On the other hand, the visual-X–ray group learned nothing despite the fact that they had a perfectly good visual cue predicting the nauseous effects of X–ray. The rats in the test reacted with their hereditary bias; they readily associated the visual size cue with the peripheral insult of shock and the chemical taste cue with internal toxicosis, but they did not make the converse associations (for further reviews see Domjan, 1980; Garcia, McGowan, & Green, 1969).

Although the rats reacted according to the evolutionary perspective rather than the empirical learning theory, this does not mean that Nature overwhelmed Nurture. The Nature–Nurture dichotomy is spurious because, quite simply, you cannot have one without the other. In the *experimentus crusis,* the rats learned to make visual-shock associations more easily than visual-illness associations because they inherited brain mechanisms from ancestors selected in a world where such associations were profitable in terms of survival, and because those brain mechanisms were appropriately nurtured and exercised during their development. Nor is the law of contiguity invalidated by the fact that the rats can relate taste to nausea in one trial; the law is merely limited to the external domain of distal signals and peripheral reinforcers such as light flashes followed by foot-shock, or bells followed by food in the mouth. Taste-illness aversions are an entirely different matter, wherein the incentive value of a taste in the mouth is modified by the subsequent homeostatic effects of feeding. This incentive modification process is a form of associative learning which can easily span CS–US intervals of several hours. To some (Logue, 1979) this seems to be a mere parametric difference, but a thousandfold difference has important practical and theoretical implications.

THE PSYCHOBIOLOGY OF EMESIS AND AVERSIONS

It is clear from the preceding discussion that when an organism becomes ill, for example as a result of exposure to radiation, its eating behavior can be disrupted. Following this period of illness, eating behavior can again be disrupted by certain stimuli that had been associated with the original illness experience, for example by tastes or smells. This observation has important implications for modern cancer treatments. Nausea and emesis are frequent side effects of treatments whose aim is to destroy the rapidly proliferating cancer cells with ionizing radiation or radiomimetic chemicals. As we shall discuss in the following sections, these side effects can lead to a disruption of the nutritional homeostatic regulation of the patient by creating conditioned nausea and conditioned taste aversions for nutrients consumed hours prior to treatment.

History of Emesis in Associationism

Nutrition is such a vital process and nausea is such a potent disruption of that process that it is not surprising to discover the historic antecedents for modern psychological treatment strategies in writings of the associationistic philosophers. For example in the early sixteenth century, Juan Luis Vives, who has been called the ''Father of Modern Psychology'' (Watson, 1915), pointed out that humans could not subsist for a moment without the nourishment of life. Self-preservation, he said, forced the human to distinguish between beneficial and harmful food (Watson, 1915, p. 11). Vives described the accidental acquisition of conditioned taste aversion in terms of associative conditioning, ''When I was a boy at Valencia, I was ill of a fever. Whilst my taste was deranged, I ate cherries. For many years afterwards, whenever I tasted fruit, I not only recalled the fever but also seemed to experience it again'' (Watson, 1915, p. 339). Thus, one half century before Bacon and two centuries before Locke, the human is described as a natural creature driven by biological necessity to mechanistically acquire empirical associations by a Catholic philosopher of Jewish heritage educated in the scientific traditions of Arabic Spain.

Clearly, Vives was aware that the cause of his illness was not the cherries, nevertheless he found cherries aversive. Recently Seligman and Hager (1972) called a similar reaction the ''Sauce Bernaise syndrome.'' Discussing Seligman's conditioned aversion for Sauce Bernaise induced by illness, they point out that conditioned aversions tend to be selective; the sauce, but neither the dinner companions nor the music, became aversive.

In 169O, John Locke discussed the neural integration of taste-illness learning, and in the bargain anticipated Johannes Muller and Herman von Helmholz's Doctrine of Specific Energies of Nerves (Garcia, 1981). Locke argued that two vastly different sensations, taste and illness, arose out of the singular physical action of the same food upon two different sensory systems, namely the sensors of the palate and the sensors of the gut respectively. In addition, Locke described how the taste of honey followed by illness results in a conditioned aversion for honey and how, subsequently, the very name of honey or the mere idea of honey brings sickness and qualms to the stomach. All these same effects, he said, would occur even if the patient could not recall the original taste-illness event (Locke, 1690, p. 397). Thus it was known very early that conditioned aversions could be established in contradiction to linguistic rationalizations and in the absence of memorial representation of the association. Locke also knew that linguistic communication and mental imagery could facilitate conditioned emetic responses. And today, mental imagery guided by linguistic instruction has been developed into a sophisticated therapeutic technique to inhibit ideas of sickness resulting from conditioned stimuli associated with chemotherapy (Burish, Redd, & Carey, this volume; Redd, Burish, & Andrykowski, this volume).

History of Emesis in Biology

Nutrition, emesis and taste aversions were also major issues in natural selection for Charles Darwin and A. R. Wallace. Darwin (1871) was puzzled by the coloration and the behavior of gaudy caterpillars who displayed themselves boldly on the tips of branches where they were in plain view of birds and other insectivores. Darwin credits Wallace with providing the following hypothesis in 1866: Conspicuously-colored caterpillars are probably protected by having a nauseous taste. But taste is not enough, because if a bird is forced to sample, numerous tender caterpillars would be fatally ruptured by exploratory pecks despite their disgusting taste. Therefore, the distinctive coloration serves to signal the bird at a distance that this species of gaudy caterpillars is unpalatable. Twenty years later, Poulton (1887) reviewed the resulting research which substantiated Wallace's hypothesis. The research revealed three major principles: (1) Flavor becomes aversive when followed by toxicosis, (2) flavor becomes palatable when it is followed by reduction of hunger, (3) visual aversions are mediated by flavor and illness.

Some of this early research has been reviewed by Garcia and Hankins (1977). One observation made on pigeons and doves in 1912 parallels the conditioned emesis now studied in human patients. Riddle and Burns (1981) reported that daily administrations of yohimbine hydrocholoride caused immediate regurgitation in the birds. Several days after beginning this treatment, some of the birds began to vomit as soon as the person associated with drug treatment entered the cage and before they were captured for treatment.

In radiation research, the most effective CS was a distinctive taste. Much earlier, Darwin (1871) described the potency of taste stimuli in the toxiphobic reactions of frogs, lizards and birds saying "When the birds rejected a caterpillar, they plainly showed, by shaking their heads, and cleansing their beaks, that they were disgusted by the taste." Recently, L. P. Brower (1969) published his elegant photographs illustrating the primacy of taste in the conditioned reactions of blue jays after the birds had eaten poisonous monarch butterflies. In the report by Riddle and Burns (1931) the CS was not a taste, but rather a person who is associated with the emetic treatment by the pigeons. In a similar fashion, the clinician and the site of treatment can serve as a CS for conditioned emesis in human patients (Burish et al., this volume; Redd et al., this volume). However, as is discussed later, when visual stimuli serve as the CS more than one trial is usually needed for the learning to take place.

On the Neural Mechanisms of Emesis

Rats, pigeons, and humans react in much the same way to X–ray exposure and emetic toxins because all three species are related through a common ancestor, the salamander. In particular, rats and humans share many homologous neural structures and behavioral patterns making the rat an excellent model for many behavioral and psychological disorders afflicting nauseated human patients. During evolution, the emetic structures were already clearly differentiated in the salamander, the first vertebrate to set foot on land (see Garcia, Forthman, Quick, & White, 1984). Taste and visceral afferents project to the viscerosensory nucleus of the medulla oblongata of the salamander and the efferent fibers project to the smooth muscles of the viscera. Thus, the salamander is superbly equipped to associate taste with poison, and to inhibit ingestion accordingly.

Emesis is also organized in the mammalian medulla oblongota. It is a complex network centering in the lateral reticular formation adjacent to the nucleus solitarius, which receives afferents from the gustatory system, the visceral system and the area postrema. The latter area also receives input from the chemical trigger zone where blood-borne chemicals are monitored. Polysynaptic routes ascend to the pons, thalamus and cortex. And, inputs from most of the cortical sensory systems descend to the emetic areas. Thus the vomiting reflex can be triggered in any number of ways: by gastric upset, taste, smell, motion, apparent motion, vision, imagery or linguistic communication. Any of these stimuli can serve as a US to establish a conditioned emetic response or a conditioned taste aversion. Any illness, toxin or agent which does not engage this system, either directly or indirectly, will not produce a taste aversion. The term ''emetic center'' reflects the specific procedures used by Borison and Wang (1951; 1953) who used emetic drugs in dogs to define one function of this complex system. Since then, research has demonstrated beyond doubt that this area is also involved in the appetitive functions, as well as the aversive aspects of ingestion.

Sensations from the mouth and oral cavity are carried to the emetic complex principally by three branches of cranial nerves. The chorda tympani of the VII nerve, the lingual-tonsilar of the IX nerve and the pharygeal of the vagus (X) nerve. The first order taste afferents terminate in the rostrolateral portion of the nucleus of the tractus solitarius. The secondary fibers from the solitary nucleus ascend through the reticular formation to the pontine taste area according to Norgren and Pfaffman (1975). From the pontine taste area the taste fibers split into two separate pathways (Norgren, 1974). One pathway leads to the lateral hypothalamus, the central amygdala and other ventral forebrain regions which are known to subserve motivation and emotional functions.

The amygdala receives inputs from the ventral pathway and plays an important role in flavor aversion learning. Large experimental lesions in the amygdala produce deficits in taste-illness conditioning (Elkins, 1980; Grupp, Linseman, & Cappell, 1976; McGowan, Hankins, & Garcia, 1972). Novocaine applied locally to the amygdala just before flavor-illness conditioning will disrupt the aversion to the odor component but not to the taste component of the target flavor. The same treatment does not disrupt odor-shock learning or taste-illness learning indicating that anesthetizing the amygdala specifically disrupts the central integration of odor, taste and illness in toxiphobic conditioning (Bermudez-Rattoni, Rusiniak, & Garcia, 1983).

The second pathway from the pontine taste area courses through relays in the ventral thalamus to an area in the anterolateral neocortex where flavor is integrated (Norgren & Wolf, 1975). This area has been dubbed the gustatory neocortex (Benjamin & Akert, 1959). Here, bilateral lesions will produce deficits in the rat's memory for a prior taste aversion and in its capacity to acquire a new taste aversion (Braun, Slick, & Lorden, 1972; Kiefer & Braun, 1977). Furthermore, precise lesions in this area can disrupt the aversion to the taste component of flavor but leave the aversion to the odor component intact. As we shall see below, aversions to the odor component are potentiated by the taste component when illness is delayed. Curiously, these precise lesions of the gustatory cortex that disrupt the taste aversion do not disrupt the capacity of the taste component to potentiate the odor component of the target flavor, indicating that taste discrimination and taste potentiation of odor are subserved by different neural areas (Kiefer, Rusiniak, & Garcia, 1982).

The main neural pathway for visceral sensations, as far as taste aversions are concerned, is the vagus (X) nerve. Sensory information from the visceral cavity is carried by other nerves, but it is the vagus that carries the visceral message directly to the emetic complex. Borison and Wang (1951, 1953; Wang and Borison, 1951) demonstrated the function of this emetic route by inducing local gastric irritations with copper sulphate, a toxic agent not readily absorbed by membrane and blood. These local irritations caused vomiting in dogs, but the vomiting could be blocked with surgical vagotomies. Injection of copper sulphate into the blood continued to promote vomiting in vagotomized dogs by the vascular route to the chemical trigger zone in the area postrema. In a parallel study, Coil, Rogers, Garcia and Novin (1978) paired saccharin and copper sulphate to demonstrate that the vagal and circulatory routes to the emetic system were also involved in taste-aversion learning in the rat. Vagotomy blocked the saccharin aversion induced by intragastric and intraperitoneal injections, but did not block the aversion induced by intravenous injections in their rats. Any substance which is rapidly absorbed into tissue and capillaries, such as alcohol, will also induce aversions in vagotomized rats via the circulatory route (Kiefer, Cabral, Rusiniak, & Garcia, 1980). However, vagotomized rats always display more rapid extinction of aversions acquired via the circulatory route or aversion acquired via the vagal route before surgery (Kiefer, Rusiniak, Garcia, & Coil, 1981). Perhaps, the vagotomy severs the efferent fibers as well as the afferents of this mixed nerve thus depriving the rat of a feedback loop which facilitates the conditioned emetic response.

Psychological Awareness of Emetic Associations

The behavior of the vagotomized rat treated with intraperitoneal copper sulphate after drinking saccharin water is especially instructive. Copper sulphate irritates the end–organs of the splanchnic and spinal nerves. A rat given copper sulfate becomes lethargic and acutely distressed by handling, and clearly must be "aware" of its illness in the ordinary sense of awareness. But it does not acquire a saccharin aversion because the visceral US does not reach the emetic complex which received the gustatory CS. *This demonstrates that neither poison nor illness nor awareness, as such, are necessary or sufficient to induce a taste aversion.* Poisons such as cyanide, which produce their deadly effect by robbing the tissues of oxygen, will not induce an aversion because they do not engage the emetic mechanism (Nachman & Hartley, 1975). Allergies and discomforts of the lower digestive tract are not sufficient to induce a taste aversion (Pelchat, Grill, Rozin, & Jacobs, 1983). But nontoxic procedures, such as rotating the subject or rotating the visual environment around the subject will induce a taste aversion (Lamon, Wilson, & Leaf, 1977; Lasiter & Braun, 1981). There is a good deal of evidence that "awareness" of the emetic action is not a necessary condition for conditioned taste aversion. The cortical functions of the rat can be degraded and disrupted by general anesthesia (Roll & Smith, 1972) or by topical chemical applications (Buresova & Bures, 1973; 1974) after the CS is presented, but before the emetic US treatment is applied, and the animal will still be able to learn the taste aversion. This same procedure would severely disrupt learning to a peripheral US. It appears that the emetic US, like many brain stem homeostatic functions, can operate "below the level of awareness."

Although the procedures to establish a conditioned taste aversion are associative, the subject does not acquire an *association* between the taste CS and the illness US; rather the subject merely acquires an *aversion* for the taste CS. Whether the subject "remembers" the associative procedure or the aversive US is of little consequence; the once acceptable CS now simply tastes "bad." There is a lot of evidence that the palatability of tastes is another one of those autonomic homeostatic functions organized at the brainstem and midbrain levels that carries on when the forebrain is incapacitated. Decerebrate rats will accept palatable flavors and reject unpalatable ones displaying the same expressive behaviors as intact rats (Grill & Norgren, 1978). These animals cannot forage for food nor will they spontaneously eat and drink, but they will accept or reject what is presented to their tongues. If they are deprived of food, they will increase their ingestion of sucrose (Grill & Norgren, 1978) and if they are injected with insulin they will also increase their sucrose but not their water intake (Flynn & Grill, 1983). There is some evidence that decerebrate rats cannot acquire a conditioned taste aversion (Grill & Norgren, 1978) but it is not entirely clear whether this inability is an impairment or an absolute loss. With other training procedures, it may yet be revealed that decerebrate rats can acquire a conditioned taste aversion under favorable test circumstances. At this point, it is clear that the consummatory phase of ingestion is mediated by hindbrain mechanisms and that the forebrain plays its principal role in the appetitive foraging phase prior to actual feeding.

On Toxiphobic Conditioning to Situational Cues

Taste followed by nausea produces a conditioned taste aversion in one trial, but when the conditioned stimulus is a situational cue and vomiting is the conditioned response, conditioning seems to require several trials. Riddle and Burns (1931) reported that two or three trials were needed before their pigeons displayed conditioned vomiting to the person associated with treatment. Redd and Andrykowski (1982) reported that conditioned emesis in cancer chemotherapy patients appears after the fourth or fifth treatment escalating in severity during subsequent treatments. In spite of the different drugs used, the description of the gradual development of conditioned vomiting is remarkably similar for pigeons and human cancer patients though the reviews describing those phenomena are separated by half a century. Garcia, Kimeldorf and Hunt (1956) reported that sham-radiation procedures produced conditioned depressions in food and water intake after three to five (75r) exposures to gamma rays in an experimental situation where distinctive taste cues were not used, so rats appear to be similar to pigeons and humans in this regard.

Best, Best, & Henggeler (1977) summarized the theoretical status, up to 1976, of the spread of conditioned nausea to stimuli other than taste. They concluded that taste and ingestinal cues are the most effective CSs, but with repeated trials, situational cues can also serve as CSs to elicit conditioned nausea. Once conditioning to one CS is strongly established, the presence of that CS will block conditioning to a second stimulus in the same situation (Kamin, 1969). For example, ingestinal cues such as taste, which are more powerfully conditioned by nausea, can block conditioning to situational cues. However, the taste cue itself can serve as an aversive agent in second–order conditioning. Garcia, Clarke and Hankins (1973) described the second-order process as follows: In the first–order, taste becomes disgusting when it is followed by emetic toxicosis, then in the second-order, situational cues become aversive because they are associated with the disgusting taste. For example, the chemotherapy patient might first become aversively conditioned to a distinctly flavored drink associated with treatment, and then secondarily become aversively conditioned to the situation in which the now aversive drink is consumed.

On Potentiation of Situational Cues by Taste and Emesis

In 1976, two novel research findings dramatically changed the pre-1976 theoretical notions discussed in the preceding section about blocking and second–order conditioning. First, Linda Brett demonstrated that taste did not block conditioning to visual cues in birds (Brett, Hankins, & Garcia, 1976). To the contrary, taste actually facilitated conditioning to visual cues. Two red-tailed hawks, which repeatedly consumed white mice as part of their normal diet were presented with a novel black mouse followed by an emetic treatment. Although black mice presumably tasted the same as the white mice, having been reared on the same food in the same laboratory, their coat-colors provided a striking visual cue. However, the keen-eyed hawks made no discriminatory use of coat-color. After three black mouse-poison trials, they refused to eat any mice, black or white. Two other hawks were given black mice marked by a mild taste cue. These birds learned to avoid black mice after one trial, at a distance, based on visual cues. Like Darwin's birds, they plainly showed by glancing at the black mouse and "smacking" their beaks that the color reminded them of the taste and made them feel sick again. Moreover, they continued to eat white mice avidly demonstrating a fine visual discrimination. This learning occurred in a single trial, so it was not second-order conditioning. It was single-order compound-cue conditioning precisely where blocking of visual cues by taste would be expected.

In the same year, Ken Rusiniak (1976) demonstrated a similar phenomenon in rats which he labeled "synergistic potentiation of odor by taste." Odor used alone proved to be poor CS for lithium injections delayed until 30 minutes after presentation of almond-scented water. Taste, used alone, proved to be a powerful CS. According to classical theory, odor and taste used together should have resulted in blocking of odor by taste, but again, the opposite happened; the taste component so facilitated conditioning to the odor component that when each component was subsequently tested alone, odor proved to be more potent than taste. The taste component was also aversive but no more so than taste used alone. In other words, the potentiation effect is asymetrical: Taste facilitates odor-illness conditioning but odor does not facilitate taste-illness conditioning. Furthermore, second-order conditioning, in which a neutral odor was paired repeatedly with a conditioned aversive taste, proved to be completely ineffective (Rusiniak, Hankins, Garcia, & Brett, 1979).

A more recent series of experiments reveals that the animal's expectation, guided by the evolutionary wisdom encoded in neural structures, also controls its conditioned associations. The experimental arrangement was a simple one. Thirsty rats routinely drank water from a spout protruding through a nose cone in a sound-attenuated chamber. Licking was recorded. On the conditioning day, a novel odor was placed in the nose cone and the rats were punished in one of two ways for drinking from the scented spout; half the animals received a mild footshock immediately after licking the scented spout and the remainder was given a nauseating (lithium-chloride) intubation 30 minutes after drinking. The shocked animals developed a fear of the odor as evidence by decreased drinking from the scented spout, but the poisoned animals continued to drink, demonstrating no aversive reactions to the scented spout. Another group of rats was treated exactly the same way except that a novel taste was added to the water at the same time that the novel odor was placed in the nose cone. Subsequently, these rats were tested with odor alone as were the other rats, but the results were in the opposite direction. The shocked animals did not fear to drink from the scented spout but the poisoned animals displayed an aversion for the odor (Rusiniak, Palmerino, Rice, Forthman, & Garcia, 1982).

To understand what happened one must view the rat intuitively and ethologically rather than objectively and behavioristically. Rats are timid animals and when they encounter a novel odor they must determine the significance of that odor for their survival. The rat finding the same familiar tasting water in the spout "attributes" the novel odor to an external source, thus it associates the odor to the peripheral insult of shock to the feet. In its ancestral memory, odor and immediate cutaneous pain are natural components of a predatory attack, and subsequently the rat responds to that odor with the defensive pawing and biting usually directed at adversaries and predators. The rat finding a novel taste in the spout in conjunction with the novel odor "attributes" the odor to the water, thus it associates the odor with the delayed internal nausea. In the ancestral memory banks, odor followed immediately by taste and later by gut-referred malaise are components of a toxic feeding bout and subsequently the rat responds to that odor by gaping and thrusting out its tongue as it naturally does to eject tainted food from the mouth (Garcia, Forthman, & White, in press).

The Rusiniak–Brett effect was substantiated by numerous studies reporting similar effects; we will comment on only a few which extended their findings in a significant way. Food color used alone is not an effective CS for a toxic US in rats, but if the colored food also has a distinctive taste, that taste will potentiate the color cue, so that the rat avoids the food on the basis of the visual cue (Galef & Osborne, 1978). Similarly in pigeons, blue water, an ineffective cue when used alone, was potentiated by the addition of taste (Clarke, Westbrook, & Irwin, 1979). Lett (in press) reviewed these phenomena and reported on her comparative studies of potentiation in avian species. In general, she finds potentiation in most species. However, seed-eaters, such as quail and pigeons, are so adept at using visual cues to select their food that when visual cues are the target stimuli it is difficult to demonstrate any improvement due to taste potentiation.

Seed-eaters, whose food is enclosed in a relatively tasteless seed-coat, have presumably developed a capacity to form direct visual-illness associations without taste mediation. However, seed-eaters do not make such effective use of visual cues to select water. For example, when seed-eating birds are tested with colored water, potentiation of visual cues by taste can be demonstrated. Garcia and Rusiniak (1980) also reviewed potentiation in a paper entitled, "What the nose learns from the mouth." This paper, which deals with "what the bird's eye learns from its beak" as well, presents an adaptive theory of potentiation.

CONCLUSION: IMPLICATIONS FOR CANCER PATIENTS

Potentiation of Conditioned Nausea in Humans

Perhaps the most interesting observation on taste potentiation of situation cues was made on human patients in the cancer chemotherapy clinic. Nerenz, Leventhal, Love, Coons and Ringler (1982) identified a potentiation reaction which is also discussed by Redd and Andrykowski (1982). According to the latter, "Patients who reported strong taste sensations during [chemotherapy] injections tended to develop anticipatory nausea/emesis which was elicited by specific stimuli in the treatment setting (e.g., needles, odor of rubbing alcohol)." It is well known that drugs injected intravenously can be tasted by human patients. Furthermore, conditioned aversions to injected substances have been reported in animals (Bradley & Mistretta, 1971). The taste of the injected drug potentiated the odor cues (rubbing alcohol) and the visual cues (needles) in the human clinic precisely as the addition of taste had potentiated odor and visual cues when the Rusiniak-Brett effect was demonstrated in the conditioning laboratory.

A second pattern of conditioned nausea was also reported by Nerenz et al. (1982) and is discussed by Redd and Andrykowski (1982) as follows: "Patients who reported both strong taste sensations and anxiety displayed a more diffuse form of anticipatory nausea/emesis. Their nausea occurred during periods of time prior to clinical visits." Thus, it appears that mental states such as anxiety and fear can effect the spread of conditioned nausea to other cues. Our research with animals supports this notion as well, a poisoned rat subsequently avoids the taste cues associated with its illness while a rat made wary and fearful by electric foot-shock avoids the auditory and visual cues associated with its pain (Garcia, Hankins, & Rusiniak, 1974; Garcia & Koelling, 1966).

Furthermore, when conditioned nausea in human patients is blocked by suggestion and guided imagery, the suggestions are usually related to images and sensations which are components of the external coping mechanisms. For example, the patients imagery may be focused on a day at the beach where the sun and sand caress the skin and the motor system is completely relaxed. These external images and exercises block out the internal concerns with the emetic system (Burish, Redd, & Carey, this volume; Redd, Burish, & Andrykowski, this volume). The same antagonistic interaction between the external coping mechanisms and the internal regulatory mechanisms can be seen in the odor-conditioning experiments with laboratory rats described earlier (Rusiniak et al., 1982). When the novel odor is associated with external shock and the CR is a motor coping response, the association of odor with internal nausea was blocked as if the odor cue had been sequestered in the external defense system where it was not available for hedonic adjustment by delayed toxic feedback. On the other hand, when odor was accompanied by taste, the odor-illness aversion was facilitated and the association with foot-shock was disrupted as if the odor cue had been stored in the feeding system where it was not available for association with external insults.

Generalizing From Human to Rat

Perhaps the most valuable function performed by this volume is the complete integration of research on animals and humans and the complete elimination of the distinction between basic and applied research. Traditionally clinicians are presumed to be applying basic techniques developed in animals to human problems. But a study of history reveals the reverse is also true. Basic facts on the visual perception of X–rays were first introspectively reported by humans and later these facts were applied to animals. Emesis was analyzed introspectively by Juan Luis Vives and John Locke before its impact upon animal behavior caught the attention of Charles Darwin and A. R. Wallace. In this volume several authors moved easily from human to rat and back again. For example, Bernstein (1978) has reported on learned taste aversions in children receiving chemotherapy after eating distinctly flavored ice cream, and Bernstein and Treneer (this volume) discuss how certain tumors that suppress appetite act as a US in the acquisition of flavor aversions. The scope and the limits of such generalizations are also discussed by Smith, Blumsack, and Bilek (this volume).

For many social and personality disorders treated in the psychotherapeutic situation, the rat appears to be a poor model because it cannot talk. No animal does, not even the chimpanzees who have been trained to use sign language or to punch out "verbal commands" on a computer terminal, because no animal possesses the specialized brain structures which produce linguistic functions. Human language is a species-specific behavior that manifests itself in human infants as a selective attention to human vocalizations and a readiness to respond verbally. Given even casual verbal feedback from other humans, the human infant learns to talk effortlessly. The best that the chimpanzee, a marvelously intelligent animal, can do is to perform some sequential discriminations rationally based on definitions of linguistic functions. And even this requires the expenditure of a lot of time and energy on the part of the trainer and the chimpanzee. The absence of homologous linguistic structures means that generalizations from other animals to humans along linguistic dimensions are impossible. But it is probably valid to generalize in the other direction, that is, to use the human's introspective descriptions to infer the existence of psychological states in animals. Rat and human possess homologous emetic structures, so we suspect that a dizzy rat, retching and displaying visual nystagmus after rotation, feels as nauseous to its stomach as a human reports verbally under the same circumstances. It may be impossible to prove, but it is a good working assumption. In research, a good working assumption is infinitely more useful than a host of rational proofs.

ACKNOWLEDGMENTS

This research was supported by the following: USPHS Program Project Grant HDO5958 and National Institute of Health Grant NS11618.

REFERENCES

Altman, J. (1975). Effects of interference with cerebellar maturation on the development of locomotion. An experimental model of neurobehavioral retardation. In N. A. Buchwald & M. A. B. Brazier (Eds.). *Mechanisms in mental retardation*. New York: Academic Press.

Baker, G. F. (Ed.). (1899). *Rontgen rays* (pp. 3–4, 7, 39–40). London: Harper Bros.

Benjamin, R. M., & Akert, K. (1959). Cortical and thalamic area–involved in taste discrimination in the albino rat. *Journal of Comparative Neurology, 111*, 260.

Bermudez-Rattoni, F., Rusiniak, K. W., & Garcia, J. (1983). Flavor-illness aversions: Potentiation of odor by taste is disrupted by application of novocaine into amygdala. *Behavioral and Neural Biology, 37*, 61–75.

Bernstein, I. L. (1978). Learned taste aversions in children receiving chemotherapy. *Science, 200*, 1302–1303.

Best, P. J., Best, M. R., & Henggeler, S. (1977). The contribution of environmental non-ingestive cues in conditioning with aversive internal consequences. In L. M. Barker, M. R. Best, & M. Domjan (Eds.), *Learning mechanisms in food selection*. Waco, Texas: Baylor University Press.

Boring, E. G. (1950). *A history of experimental psychology*. New York: Appleton-Century-Crofts.

Borison, H. L., & Wang, S. C. (1951). Copper sulphate emesis: A study of afferent pathways from the gastrointestinal tract. *American Journal of Physiology, 164*, 520–526.

Borison, H. L., & Wang, S. C. (1953). Physiology and pharmacology of vomiting. *Pharmacological Review, 5*, 193–230.

Bradley, R. M., & Mistretta, C. (1971). Intravascular taste in rats as demonstrated by conditioned aversion to sodium saccharin. *Journal of Comparative and Physiological Psychology, 75*, 186–189.

Braun, J. J., Slick, T. B., & Lorden, J. F. (1972). Involvement of gustatory neocortex in the learning of taste aversions. *Physiology and Behavior, 9*, 637–641.

Brett, L. P., Hankins, W. G., & Garcia, J. (1976). Prey-lithium aversions: III Buteo hawks. *Behavioral Biology, 17*, 87–89.

Brower, L. P. (1969). Ecological chemistry. *Scientific American, 220*, 22–29.

Brown, P. (1936). *American martyrs to science through the Roentgen rays* (pp. 6–7, 91–92, 100–105, 148) Baltimore: Charles C. Thomas.

Buchwald, N. A., Garcia, J., Feder, B. H., & Bach-y-Rita, G. (1964). Ionizing radiation as a perceptual and aversive stimulus. II. Electrophysiological studies. In T. J. Haley & R. S. Snyder (Eds.), *The second international symposium on the responses of the nervous system to ionizing radiation* (pp. 688–699). Boston: Little, Brown, and Company.

Buresova, O., & Bures, J. (1973). Cortical and subcortical components of the conditioned saccharin aversion. *Physiology and Behavior, 11,* 435–439.

Buresova, O., & Bures, J. (1974). Functional decortication in the CS–US interval decrease efficiency of taste aversion learning. *Behavioral Biology, 12,* 357–364.

Chaddock, T. E. (1972). Visual detection of X–ray by the rhesus monkey. *Journal of Comparative and Physiological Psychology, 78,* 190–201.

Clarke, J. C., Westbrook, R. F., & Irwin, J. (1979). Potentiation instead of overshadowing in the pigeon. *Behavioral and Neural Biology, 25,* 18–29.

Codman, E. A. (1901). No practical danger from the X–ray. *Boston Medical and Surgical Journal, 144*(5), 197.

Cooper, G. P. (1968). Receptor origin of the olfactory bulb response to ionizing radiation. *American Journal of Physiology, 215,* 803–806.

Coil, J. D., Rogers, R. C., Garcia, J., & Novin, D. (1978). Conditioned taste aversions: Vagal and circulatory mediation of the toxic unconditioned stimulus. *Behavioral Biology, 24,* 509–519.

Compton, A. H. (1935). *X–rays in theory and experiment* (p. 1). New York: D. van Nostrand & Company.

D'Arcy, F. J., & Porter, N. A. (1962). Detection of cosmic ray u-mesons by the human eye. *Nature, 196,* 1013–1014.

Darwin, C. (1871). *The decent of man and selection in relation to sex.* London: Murray.

Domjan, M. (1980). Ingestinal learning: Unique and general processes. In J. S. Rosenblatt, R. A. Hinde, C. Beer, & M. C. Busnel (Eds.), *Advances in the study of behavior* (Vol. 2). New York: Academic Press.

Elkins, R. L. (1980). Attenuation of X–ray induced taste aversions by the olfactory bulb or amygdaloid lesion. *Physiology and Behavior, 24,* 515–521.

Eisner, T., & Grant, R. P. (1981). Toxicity, odor aversion, and "olfactory aposematism." *Science, 213,* 476.

Estes, W. K., & Skinner, B. F. (1941). Some quantitative properties of anxiety. *Journal of Experimental Psychology, 29,* 390–400.

Flynn, F. W., & Grill, H. J. (1983). Insulin elicits ingestion in decerebrate rats. *Science, 221,* 188–189.

Galef, B. G., & Osborne, B. (1978). Novel taste facilitation of the association of visual cues with toxicosis in rats. *Journal of Comparative and Physiological Psychology, 92,* 907–916.

Garcia, J. (1981). Tilting at the papermills of academe. *American Psychologist, 36*(2), 149–158.

Garcia, J., Buchwald, N. A., Bach-y-rita, G., Feder, B. H., & Koelling, R. A. (1963). Electroencephalographic responses to ionizing radiation. *Science, 140,* 289–290.

Garcia, J., Buchwald, N. A., Feder, B. H., & Koelling, R. A. (1962). Immediate detection of X–rays by the rat. *Nature, 196,* 1014–1015.

Garcia, J., Buchwald, N. A., Feder, B. H., Koelling, R. A., & Tedrow, L. (1964). Sensitivity of the head to X–ray. *Science, 144,* 1470–1472.

Garcia, J., Buchwald, N. A., Hull, C. D., & Koelling, R. A. (1964). Adaptive responses to ionizing radiations. *Bol. Inst. Estud. Med. Biol. Mex., 22,* 101–113.

Garcia, J., Clarke, J. C., & Hankins, W. G. (1973). Natural responses to scheduled rewards. In P. Bateson & P. Klopfer (Eds.), *Perspectives in ethology,* New York: Plenum Press.

Garcia, J., Ervin, F. R., & Koelling, R. A. (1966). Learning with prolonged delay of reinforcement. *Psychonomic Science, 5,* 121–122.

Garcia, J., Ervin, F. R., & Koelling, R. A. (1967). Toxicity of serum from irradiated donors. *Nature, 213*, 682–683.

Garcia, J., Forthman, Quick, D., & White, B. (1984). Conditioned disgust and fear from mollusk to monkey. In D. L. Alkon & J. Farley (Eds.), *Primary neural substrates of learning and behavioral change* (pp. 47–61). New York: Cambridge University Press.

Garcia, J., Green, K. F., & McGowan, B. K. (1969). X-ray as an olfactory stimulus. In C. Pfaffman (Ed.), *Taste and olfaction III* (pp. 299–309). New York: Rockefeller University Press.

Garcia, J., & Hankins, W. G. (1977). On the origin of food aversion paradigms. In L. M. Barker, M. Domjan & M. Best (Eds.), *Learning mechanisms in food selection*, Waco, Texas: Baylor University Press.

Garcia, J., Hankins, W. G., & Rusiniak, K. W. (1974). Behavioral regulation of the milieu interne in man and rat. *Science, 185*, 824–831.

Garcia, J., & Kimeldorf, D. J. (1960). Some factors which influence radiation conditioned behavior in rats. *Radiation Research, 68*, 383–395.

Garcia, J., Kimeldorf, D. J., & Hunt, E. L. (1956). Conditioned responses to manipulative procedures resulting from exposure to gamma radiation. *Radiological Research, 5*, 79–87.

Garcia, J., Kimeldorf, D. J., & Hunt, E. L. (1957). Spatial avoidance behavior in the rat as a result of exposure to ionizing radiation. *British Journal of Radiology, 30*, 318–321.

Garcia, J., Kimeldorf, D. J., & Hunt, E. L. (1961). The use of ionizing radiation as a motivating stimulus. *Psychological Review, 68*, 383–395.

Garcia, J., Kimeldorf, D. J., & Koelling, R. A. (1955). Conditioned aversion to saccharin resulting from exposure to gamma radiation. *Science, 122*, 157–158.

Garcia, J., & Koelling, R. A. (1967). A comparison of aversions induced by X-rays, drugs and toxins. *Radiation Research Supplement, 7*, 439–450.

Garcia, J., & Koelling, R. A. (1966). Relation of cue to consequence in avoidance learning. *Psychonomic Science, 4*, 123–124.

Garcia, J., & Koelling, R. A. (1971). The use of ionizing rays as a mammalian olfactory stimulus. In L. M. Beidler (Ed.), *Handbook of sensory physiology* (Vol. 4), *chemical senses* (pp. 449–464). New York: Springer-Verlag.

Garcia, J., McGowan, B. K., Ervin, F. R., & Koelling, R. A. (1968). Cues: Their relative effectiveness as a function of the reinforcer. *Science, 160*, 794–795.

Garcia, J., McGowan, B. K., & Green, K. F. (1969). Biological constraints on conditioning. In A. Black & W. Prokasy (Eds.), *Classical conditioning* (pp. 3–27). Hamilton, Ontario: McMaster University Press.

Garcia, J., & Rusiniak, K. W. (1980). What the nose learns from the mouth. In D. Muller-Schwarze & P. M. Silverstein (Eds.), *Chemical signals*. New York: Plenum Press.

Grill, H. J., & Norgren, R. (1978). The taste reactivity test. I. Mimetic responses to gustatory stimuli in neurologically normal rats. *Brain Research, 143*, 263.

Grupp, L. A., Linseman, M. A., & Cappell, H. (1976). Effects of amygdala lesions on taste aversions produced by amphetamine and LiCl. *Pharmacology, Biochemistry and Behavior, 4*, 541–544.

Hull, C. D., Garcia, J., Buchwald, N. A., Dubrowsky, B., & Feder, B. H. (1965). The role of the olfactory system in arousal to X-ray. *Nature, 205*, 627–628.

Hunt, E. L., Carrol, H. W., & Kimeldorf, D. J. (1968). Effects of dose and partial body exposure on conditioning through radiation induced factor. *Physiology and Behavior, 3*, 809–813.

Hunt, E. L., & Kimeldorf, D. J. (1962). Evidence for direct stimulation of the mammalian nervous system with ionizing radiation. *Science, 137*, 857–859.

Hunt, E. L., & Kimeldorf, D. J. (1964). Behavioral arousal and neural activation as radiosensitive reactions. *Radiation Research, 21*, 91–110.

Kamin, L. J. (1969). Predictability, surprise, attention and conditioning. In B. Campbell & R. Church (Eds.), *Punishment and aversive behavior*. New York: Appelton-Century Crofts.

Kiefer, S. W., & Braun, J. J. (1977). Absence of differential associative responses to novel and familiar taste stimuli in rats lacking gustatory neocortex. *Journal of Comparative and Physiological Psychology, 91,* 498–507.

Kiefer, S. W., Cabral, R. J., Rusiniak, K. W., & Garcia, J. (1980). Ethanol-induced aversions in rats with subdiaphramatic vagotomies, *Behavioral and Neural Biology, 29,* 246.

Kiefer, S. W., Rusiniak, K. W., & Garcia, J. (1982). Flavor-illness aversions: Potentiation of odor by taste in rats with gustatory neocortex ablations. *Journal of Comparative and Physiological Psychology, 96,* 540–548.

Kiefer, S. W., Rusiniak, K. W., Garcia, & Coil, J. D. (1981). Vagotomy facilitates extinction of conditioned taste aversions in rats. *Journal of Comparative and Physiology Psychology, 95,* 114–122.

Kimeldorf, D. J., & Hunt, E. L. (1965). *Ionizing radiation: Neural function and behavior.* New York: Academic Press.

Lamon, S., Wilson, G. T., & Leaf, R. C. (1977). Human classical aversion conditioning: Nausea versus electric shock in the reduction of large beverage consumption. *Behavioral Research and Therapy, 15,* 313.

Lasiter, P. S., & Braun, J. J. (1981). Shock facilitation of taste aversion learning. *Behavioral and Neural Biology, 32,* 277–281.

Lett, B. T. (in press). Taste potentiation in poison avoidance learning. In M. L. Commons, R. J. Herrnstein, & A. R. Wagner (Eds.), *Quantitative analyses of behavior: Vol. 3, acquisition.* Cambridge: Ballinger.

Levy, C. K., Ervin, F. R., & Garcia, J. (1970). The effect of serum from irradiated donors on gastrointestinal function. *Nature, 225,* 463–464.

Levy, C. J., Carroll, M. E., Smith, J. C., & Hofer, K. G. (1974). Antihistamines block radiation induced taste aversions. *Science, 186,* 1044–1046.

Lipetz, L. E. (1955). The X–ray and radium phosphines. *British Journal of Opthamalogy, 39,* 577–598.

Locke, J. (1975). *An essay concerning human understanding,* P. H. Nidditch (Ed.). Oxford: Clarendon Press. (Originally published 1690.)

Logue, A. W. (1979). Taste aversion and the generality of the laws of learning. *Psychological Bulletin, 86,* 276–296.

McGowan, B. K., Hankins, W. G., & Garcia, J. (1972). Limbic lesions and control of the internal and external environment. *Behavioral Biology, 7,* 841–852.

Muncheryan, H. M. (1940). *Modern physics of roentgenology* (p. 215). Los Angeles: Wetzel Publishing Company.

Nachman, M., & Hartley, P. L. (1975). The role of illness in producing taste aversion in rats: A comparison of several rodenticides. *Journal of Comparative and Physiological Psychology, 89,* 101–1018.

Nerenz, D. R., Leventhal, H., Love, R. R., Coons, H., & Ringler, K. (1982). *The development of anticipatory nausea during cancer chemotherapy.* Unpublished manuscript, Madison: University of Wisconsin.

Newell, R. R., & Borley, W. E. (1941). Roentgen measurement of visual acuity in cataractous eyes. *Radiology, 37,* 54–61.

Norgren, R. (1974). Gustatory afferents to ventral forebrain. *Brain Research, 81,* 285.

Norgren, R., & Pfaffman, C. (1975). The pontine taste area in the rat. *Brain Research, 91,* 99.

Norgren, R., & Wolf, G. (1975). Projections of the thalamic gustatory and lingual areas in the rat. *Brain Research, 92,* 123–129.

Pelchat, M. L., Grill, H. J., Rozin, P., & Jacobs, J. (1983). Quality of acquired responses to tastes by Rattus norvegicus depends on type of associated discomfort. *Journal of Comparative Psychology, 92,* 140–153.

Pinsky, L. S., Osborne, W. Z., Bailey, J. V., Benson, R. E., & Thompson, L. F. (1974). Light flashes observed by astronauts on Apollo 11 through 17. *Science, 183*, 957–959.

Poulton, E. G. (1887). The experimental proof of the protective value of color and marking in insects in reference to their vertebrate enemies. *Proceedings of the Zoological Society of London*, pp. 191–274.

Redd, W. H., & Andrykowski, M. A. (1982). Behavioral intervention in cancer treatment: Controlling aversion reactions to chemotherapy. *Journal of Consulting Clinical Psychology, 50*, 1018–1029.

Riddle, O., & Burns, F. H. (1931). A conditioned emetic reflex in the pigeon. *Proceedings of the Society for Experimental Biology and Medicine, 5629*, 979–981.

Roll, D. L., & Smith, J. C. (1972). Conditioned taste aversion in anesthetized rats. In M. E. P. Seligman & J. L. Hager, *Biological boundaries of learning* (pp. 98–102). New York: Appleton-Century-Crofts.

Rollins, W. (1903). *Notes on X–light* (pp. 174–177, 192). Cambridge: Cambridge University Press.

Rugh, R. (1962). Major radiological concepts and effects of ionizing radiations on the embryo and fetus. In T. J. Haley & R. S. Snyder (Eds.), *Response of the nervous system to ionizing radiation*. New York: Academic Press.

Rusiniak, K. W. (1976). *Roles of olfaction and taste in appetitive and consummatory behavior during illness aversion conditioning*. Unpublished doctoral dissertation, University of California, Los Angeles.

Rusiniak, K. W., Hankins, W. G., Garcia, J. & Brett, L. P. (1979). Flavor-illness aversions: Potentiation of odor by taste in rats. *Behavioral and Neural Biology, 25*, 1–17.

Rusiniak, K. W., Palmerino, C. C., Rice, A. G., Forthman, D. L., & Garcia, J. (1982). Flavor-illness aversions: Potentiation of odor by taste with toxin but not shock in rats. *Journal of Comparative and Physiological Psychology, 96*(4), 527–539.

Sahakian, W. S. (1968). *History of psychology: A sourcebook in systematic psychology* (pp. 143–144). Itasca, IL: F. E. Peacock Publishers.

Seligman, M. E. P., & Hager, J. L. (1972). *Biological boundaries of learning*. Englewood Cliffs, NJ: Prentice-Hall.

Testa, T. J. (1974). Causal relationships and the aquisition of avoidance responses. *Psychological Review, 81*(6), 491–505.

Thompson, S. P. (1921). *Light visible and invisible*. London: Macmillan and Co.

Wang, S. C., & Borison, H. L. (1951). The vomiting center: A critical experimental analysis. *Archives of Neural Psychology, 63*, 928.

Watson, F. (1915). The father of modern psychology. *Psychological Review, 22*, 333–353.

3 Specific Taste Preferences: An Alternative Explanation for Eating Changes in Cancer Patients*

Neil E. Grunberg
Department of Medical Psychology
Uniformed Services University of the Health Sciences

INTRODUCTION AND BACKGROUND

For many people the word "cancer" brings to mind an emaciated patient struggling painfully and weakly through daily tasks. The syndrome of weight loss and malnourishment which is common for some cancers, such as lung and liver, is known as "cachexia." Although it appears in many cancer patients, it is little understood. As recently as 1981, Buzby and Steinberg wrote: "The etiology of cachexia in most cancer patients is not known. No simple unifying explanation can account for the tissue wasting seen in all patients. Rather, several factors acting simultaneously or sequentially to varying degrees produce the common end result of cancer cachexia" (Buzby & Steinberg, 1981, p. 692).

Cancer cachexia does not accompany all cancers. This fact is relevant to attempts to understand the mechanisms underlying this physical wasting away and to efforts to alleviate or attenuate the cachexia. Because cachexia does not accompany all cancers, careful examination and comparison of when it does and does not occur (e.g., which cancers, what stages of cancer) may provide insight into the causes of cancer cachexia. In addition, it is important to recognize that the cachexia may result both from the cancer itself and from some treatments, including chemotherapy and radiotherapy (e.g., Costa & Donaldson, 1979). Cachexia contributes to mortality (i.e., cachexia itself often is the cause of death), affects quality of life, and alters the effectiveness of responses to some

*The opinions or assertions contained herein are the private ones of the author and are not to be construed as official or reflecting the views of the DoD or the USUHS.

treatments. For all of these reasons, cachexia is a phenomenon which warrants intensive study.

Cachexia results from both physiological and psychological causes.[1] The physiological include metabolic, endocrinologic, and biochemical factors. Physiological factors which contribute to the cachexic response to tumors are discussed particularly well by Buzby and Steinberg (1981), Costa (1963), Morrison (1979), Waterhouse (1963), and Young (1977). Physiological factors which are involved in the cachexic response to cancer treatment, including chemotherapy, immunotherapy, radiotherapy, and surgery, are discussed by Donaldson (1977), Donaldson and Lenon (1979), Ohnuma and Holland (1977), and Shils (1979). These factors mostly involve changes in energy utilization. That is, tumorigenesis or cancer treatments act through physiological effects to increase the rate at which calories are used in some cancer patients and thereby result in malnourishment and a decrease in body weight.

Psychological and behavioral factors contribute to cancer cachexia mostly by decreasing energy (caloric) intake. These factors include mental and emotional state (e.g., depression), mechanical effects which are not related to hunger or taste (e.g., changes in ability to chew depending on the site of the tumor), and direct changes in eating behavior. The focus of this chapter is on eating and cachexia. Therefore, the other factors cited above (i.e., physiological factors and psychological factors other than eating per se) which contribute to cancer cachexia are not discussed further.

Within the topic of "eating changes," distinctions must be made between "anorexia" and "decreased food consumption." Anorexia literally means a decrease in appetite. It also is used more loosely to refer to decreased food consumption. However, these are two distinct phenomena. They may occur together or one may occur without the other. The mechanisms which alter the hunger drive and therefore affect appetite may or may not play a role in decreasing food consumption per se. For example, a person who does not "have an appetite," may eat tremendous amounts of food prepared by a favorite aunt or available at a single price, all-you-can-eat, smorgasbord buffet. A hungry dieter, in contrast, who maintains restraint, will limit food consumption in these situations. Whether cachexic cancer patients have changes in appetite, changes in food consumption, or both must be clearly delineated if the contribution of decreased energy intake to cachexia is to be understood and treated. This chapter will concentrate on changes in food consumption that do not necessarily involve changes in hunger.

[1]For expositional clarity a marked distinction is drawn between physiological and psychological causes. These classifications are not meant to indicate or to imply a philosophical dualism. Instead, these terms are used to distinguish between causes that are mostly biological in mechanistic and common sense ways (e.g., metabolic changes) and causes that are largely behavioral (e.g., eating changes) or psychological (e.g., changes in affect).

BIOBEHAVIORAL EXPLANATIONS OF CHANGES IN FOOD CONSUMPTION IN CANCER PATIENTS

Two major biobehavioral explanations have been offered to account for changes in food consumption in response to tumorigenesis and cancer treatment: (1) learned taste aversion; and (2) taste acuity changes. The phenomenon of learned taste aversion is well documented (e.g., Garcia, Hankins, & Rusiniak, 1974, Garcia, Kimeldorf, & Koelling, 1955; Garcia & Koelling, 1967). The historical roots and a review of the phenomenon are discussed in some detail in this volume by Robertson and Garcia. More recently, it has been demonstrated that taste-aversion learning occurs in animals and humans in response to tumor growth and cancer chemotherapy (e.g., Bernstein, 1978; Bernstein & Bernstein, 1981; Bernstein & Sigmundi, 1980; Bernstein, Vitiello, & Sigmundi, 1980; Bernstein, Wallace, Bernstein, Bleyer, Chard, & Hartmann, 1979; Smith & Blumsack, 1981). Cancer-related learned taste aversion and its potential contribution to cancer cachexia is discussed in this volume by Bernstein and Treneer and by Smith, Blumsack, & Bilek. It is worth noting here that learned taste aversions may contribute to decreased food consumption in cancer patients. However, for reasons discussed in this chapter, learned taste aversions cannot be the sole explanation for changes in energy intake in cancer patients.

The other explanation for cancer-related eating changes, which has received substantial attention in the literature, is change in taste acuity. It has been reported that cancer patients exhibit shifts in detection and recognition taste thresholds (e.g., Chlebowski, Heber, & Block, 1981; DeWys, 1978; DeWys, Costa, & Henkin, 1981; DeWys & Walters, 1975; Gorshein, 1977; Hall, 1979; Mossman & Henkin, 1978; Russ & DeWys, 1978). In particular, these studies report that cancer patients have elevated taste thresholds for sweet (sucrose) and lowered taste thresholds for bitter (urea). Some investigators and clinicians have suggested that these shifts in taste thresholds (e.g., lowered urea threshold) lead to changes in food consumption (e.g., decreased consumption of meat) which result in decreased caloric intake and therefore loss of body weight (e.g., DeWys, 1979; DeWys & Walters, 1975). However, there are a number of issues and empirical findings to consider before concluding that changes in taste thresholds could actually lead to changes in food consumption. Settle, Quinn, Brand, Kare, Mullen, and Brown (1979) have reanalyzed some of the data from taste acuity studies of cancer patients (e.g., DeWys & Walters, 1975) and argue that all of the reported changes did not occur (e.g., there actually were no changes in bitter recognition thresholds). Rather, the initial analyses were incorrectly computed. This point, of course, casts serious doubt on conclusions drawn from these data that cancer and its treatment alter taste acuity. However, Settle or others have not leveled this devastating criticism against all of the taste acuity studies. In addition, Settle et al. (1979) themselves report some significant taste acuity changes. Therefore, a possible role for taste acuity changes in cancer cachexia cannot be completely dismissed on the basis of the reanalyses by Settle et al. Instead, other issues must be considered before generalizing to cancer cachexia from any taste threshold changes that do occur.

Based on empirical data, Bartoshuk (1978) has argued that taste threshold studies may not generalize to suprathreshold sensitivity. That is, the minimum concentration at which a given substance is detected by tasting it (detection threshold) or recognized by tasting it (recognition threshold) may not indicate anything about how the taste of that substance is perceived when presented in a concentration that exceeds detection and recognition thresholds (i.e., suprathreshold values), as in most foods. In fact, Bartoshuk cites examples of threshold and suprathreshold analyses providing conflicting conclusions about taste sensitivities. For instance, an individual who has a higher detection threshold (i.e., less sensitivity) for a particular substance compared to another individual, does not necessarily display higher suprathreshold values (i.e., less sensitivity to a concentration of that substance which exceeds the detection and recognition thresholds). Therefore, shifts in threshold values are not necessarily informative about changes in suprathreshold acuity, and taste threshold changes cannot be used to generalize about changes in food consumption.

Another issue that bears on the generalizability of changes in taste acuity to changes in food consumption is that taste acuity differs before and after eating (Kaplan & Powell, 1969). It must also be considered that self-reports of taste impairment are not necessarily related to actual changes in acuity (Mossman & Henkin, 1978). Also, there is evidence that taste sensitivity to liquids and solids show little correlation (Mackey & Jones, 1954). In addition, taste acuity may differ for the same tastes if those tastes are assessed in the form of different foods (Pangborn & Trabue, 1967). For all of these reasons, changes in food consumption or food preferences cannot be extrapolated from taste acuity studies. Food consumption and preferences must be measured directly.

AN ALTERNATIVE BIOBEHAVIORAL EXPLANATION OF CHANGES IN FOOD CONSUMPTION IN CANCER PATIENTS

Clinical observations indicate that cancer patients exhibit changes in taste preferences or specific food preferences. A common report is that cancer patients dislike meat (e.g., DeWys, 1977; Dudgeon, DeLisa, & Miller, 1980; Morrison, 1976, 1978; Schein, Macdonald, Waters, & Haidak, 1975). Other specific food preferences also have been noted in cancer patients. For example, DeWys and Herbst (1977) reported preferences for milk-based products compared to synthetic chemically defined nutritional products. Gormican (1980) also reported that many cancer patients preferred cold dairy products. Aker (1979) reported that bone marrow transplant patients commonly prefer ". . . cold, clear liquids such as fruit-ades, carbonated beverages, Popsicles, and Jell-O" (page 2104). In contrast, these patients do not tolerate warm broths or puddings. In a study of breast and colon cancer patients, Carson and Gormican (1977) found both increases and decreases in preferences for specific foods. Brewin (1980) examined patients attending a radiotherapy and oncology center and found increased preferences for certain foods and decreased preferences for other foods. Most of these reports lack the rigor of carefully designed empirical studies. Many different tumors and treatments are included together and controls often are lacking. The few studies that carefully measure taste preference judgments (e.g., Nielsen, Theologides, & Vickers, 1980; Settle et al., 1979) rely heavily on self-report data and do not measure actual food consumption. It is therefore difficult to come to any firm, uncontestable conclusions. Overall, these studies and clinical observations indicate that changes in taste preferences do occur in cancer patients and that these changes seem to include both decreases and increases in preferences for specific foods.

Changes in specific food preferences might be explained by learned taste aversions or changes in taste acuity. Learned taste aversions could explain decreased preferences for foods in many instances (see Bernstein & Webster; Robertson & Garcia; Smith et al., this volume). However, learned taste aversions cannot account for any increased taste preferences. Taste acuity might be involved in specific food preferences but, as already has been discussed, changes in taste acuity do not necessarily correlate with changes in food consumption. There is another aspect of conditioned taste changes that theoretically could account for increased taste preferences: conditioned taste preferences. Compared to conditioned taste aversions which are well documented and which have been repeatedly demonstrated in both humans and animals, conditioned taste preferences have received less research attention and most of the studies that have been reported do not provide unequivocal demonstrations of conditioned taste preferences (see Zahorik, 1977, for a review of this topic). There have been some recent demonstrations of conditioned taste preferences (e.g., Bolles, Hayward, & Crandall, 1981; Capaldi & Myers, 1982; Davidson-Codjoe & Holman, 1982). However, this phenomenon does not yet have the mountain of empirical support that conditioned taste aversion has.

There is an alternative explanation for changes in specific food preferences. This explanation derives in part from the phenomenon of "alliesthesia." Readers well acquainted with conditioned taste changes will recognize that some investigators argue (at least implicitly) that conditioned taste changes and alliesthesia are related. This position certainly is reasonable. However, because conditioned taste changes and alliesthesia differ on at least methodological and paradigmatic grounds, they are distinguished in this chapter.

"Alliesthesia" literally means changed (allios) sensation (esthesia). This term was coined by Cabanac (1971) to describe the phenomenon in which a particular external stimulus (e.g., a particular food) is perceived as either pleasant or unpleasant depending on the internal state of the body (the "milieu interieur"). In the case of a taste preference, hedonic judgments depend on the physiological state of the individual. For example, people report that sucrose solutions taste more pleasant after insulin injections than after saline injections (Briese & Quijada, 1979). Also, pleasant, sweet-tasting sucrose solutions become unpleasant after ingestion of glucose (Cabanac, 1971). Other studies also show that changes in physiological state affect taste pleasantness (e.g., Cabanac, Minaire, & Adair, 1968; Moskowitz, Kumraiah, Sharma, Jacobs, & Sharma, 1976). Cabanac's notion of alliesthesia as applied to eating behavior emphasizes changes in hedonic judgments and taste preferences. Other investigators and writers have extended alliesthesia to other aspects of eating and food consumption such as hunger (e.g., Thompson & Campbell, 1977) and taste thresholds (e.g., Henkin, Gill, & Bartter, 1963). In addition, alliesthesia has been used to explain specific hungers—the phenomenon in which an animal deficient in a particular nutrient selects foods which contain that nutrient, such as a craving for salt or thiamine (see Rozin & Kalat, 1971, for a detailed discussion of specific hungers).

To return to cancer-related weight changes: Are taste preference changes a reasonable alternative to learned taste aversions and taste threshold or acuity changes? Besides the papers discussed so far, there are many others which cite examples of altered taste preferences as well as altered taste thresholds (e.g., DeWys, 1974; Garattini, Bizzi, Donnelli, Guaitani, Samanin, & Spreafico, 1980; Theologides, 1977; Williams & Cohen, 1978) and altered taste preferences along with taste aversions (e.g., DeWys, 1974; Rose, 1978). However, it also has been reported recently that differences in taste preferences occur without differences in taste thresholds (Trant, Serin, & Douglass, 1982). Therefore, altered taste preferences per se seem to provide a third, distinct explanation of changes in food consumption by cancer patients. But could changes in taste preferences contribute to changes in body weight? None of the work cited above addresses this possibility. Studies of taste preferences and alliesthesia rarely examine body weight or caloric intake over a long enough period to reach any conclusions about effects of taste preferences on body weight. To answer this important question, I reviewed a series of studies that have examined the relationship between cigarette smoking and body weight. Although this topic may appear to be far afield, these studies are quite relevant and suggest an answer to the question of the potential relationships between taste preferences and body weight.

THE EFFECTS OF NICOTINE ON BODY WEIGHT, FOOD CONSUMPTION, AND TASTE PREFERENCES

Reviews of studies that have examined the relationship between cigarette smoking and body weight reveal that habitual smokers weigh less than comparably aged nonsmokers, and that habitual smokers who give up smoking gain weight (Grunberg, 1982a; Wack & Rodin, 1982). Three different explanations for this inverse relationship have been offered: smokers eat less food than do nonsmokers and ex-smokers (e.g., Birch, 1975); smoking increases energy utilization (e.g., by increasing metabolic rate) and thereby alters body weight (e.g., Comroe, 1960); ex-smokers consume increased amount of specific foods, such as sweet-tasting high caloric foods (e.g., Myrsten, Elgerot, & Edgren, 1977). The first explanation for the smoking/body weight relationship is basically the same as the psychological/behavioral (i.e., changes in food consumption) explanations that have been offered to explain cancer cachexia. The second explanation for the smoking/body weight relationship corresponds to the physiological explanation (i.e., changes in energy utilization) for cancer cachexia. The third explanation (i.e., changes in *specific* food consumption) is essentially the same as the alternative biobehavioral explanation for cancer cachexia that was described in the previous section of this chapter. Therefore, careful examination of which of these three explanations account for the effects of cigarette smoking on body weight may provide insight regarding cancer cachexia.

Until recently, there has been little research evidence in support of any one of these three basic explanations for the smoking/body weight relationship. In order to examine the two behavioral explanations, Grunberg (1982a) conducted two laboratory studies. The first study used rats to investigate the effects of nicotine administration and abstinence from nicotine on body weight, food consumption, and taste preferences. Nicotine was used for two reasons: it (or one of its metabolites) appears to be the component of tobacco which produces biological dependence on cigarettes (e.g., Russell, 1971; Schachter, 1978), and nicotine administration to animals alters body weight in a fashion analogous to the body weight changes associated with cigarette smoking (e.g., Passey, Elson, & Conners, 1961; Schechter & Cook, 1976). The second study examined the food consumption and taste preferences of human habitual smokers who were allowed to smoke, smokers who abstained from smoking, and nonsmokers. These studies were designed to determine whether changes in general food consumption or specific food consumption occurred, and whether these changes could contribute to changes in body weight.

The rat study examined the effects of nicotine administration and abstinence from nicotine on total food consumption, sweet-tasting food consumption, and body weight. Food, water, and sugar solutions were available 24 hours each day. The food was a standard laboratory chow (Ralston Purina Company Rat Chow 5012). The sugar solutions were 35%, 25%, and 10% w/v d-glucose. (The 35% and 25% sugar solutions tasted extremely sweet to humans. The 10% solution tasted only slightly sweet.) Daily measurements were made of body weight, food consumption, water consumption, and sugar solution consumption before, during, and after drug administration. The study included 20 male albino Sprague–Dawley rats. The rats were individually housed in an animal vivarium with a 12-hour light–dark cycle. These animals all weighed roughly 450 grams at the beginning of the study. After an initial gentling period, the daily measurements were made for two weeks. Then, Alzet miniosmotic pumps (model 1702) were subcutaneously implanted in each rat between the head and back. These devices deliver their contents at a rate of roughly 0.5 μl/hour for about two weeks (Theeuwes & Yum, 1977). Physiological saline was used to make the nicotine solutions (made from nicotine dihydrochloride) and was the control solution. Five animals received saline, five received 2.5 millograms of nicotine per kilogram of body weight per day, five received 5.0 mg nicotine per kg per day, and five received 10.0 mg nicotine per kg per day. The sugar solutions were removed the day before and the day of surgery and for two days afterwards to reduce the likelihood of learned taste aversions. Following surgery, daily measurements were made of body weight, food consumption, water consumption, and sugar solution consumption during drug administration (roughly two weeks) and for an additional two weeks after the minipumps were empty.

Fig. 3.1 presents the mean body weight for each experimental group before, during, and after drug administration. Before drug administration, the body weights of all four groups of rats were similar. During drug administration animals that received nicotine gained significantly less weight than did the control group (all $ps < 0.01$). After cessation of nicotine administration, animals that had received nicotine gained weight at a greater rate than did control animals. It is important to determine whether changes in general food consumption or specific food consumption accounted for the effects of nicotine on body

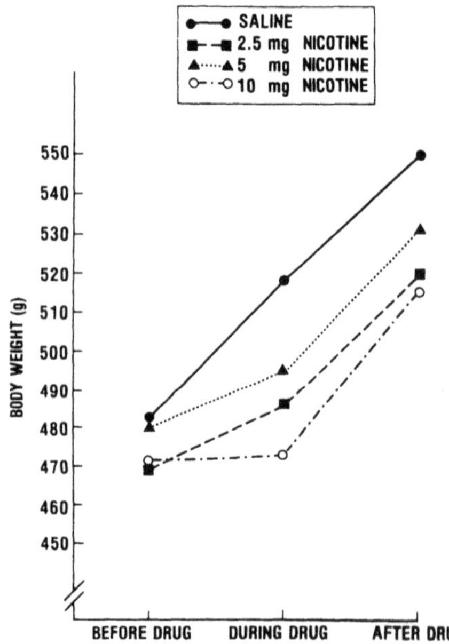

FIG. 3.1. Average body weights before, during, and after drug administration. Reprinted with permission from Grunberg, 1982a, *Addictive Behaviors*, 7, The effects of nicotine and cigarette smoking on food consumption and taste preferences, 1982, Pergamon Press, Ltd.

weight. If these behavioral factors contributed to the body weight changes, then, by analogy, they also may play a role in the weight changes of cancer patients.

An analysis of caloric intake from laboratory chow and sugar solutions revealed that animals receiving nicotine reduced their total caloric intake during drug administration and increased their total caloric intake after cessation of nicotine administration. These changes in total caloric intake were significantly different from the eating behavior of the control animals (at the 0.05 level or better for each of the nicotine groups). These changes in total caloric intake paralleled the changes in body weight and, therefore, could at least partially account for the body weight changes. Caloric intake from the bland-tasting laboratory chow and sweet-tasting sugar solutions were measured separately in order to examine general and specific food consumption.

It is apparent from Fig. 3.2 that changes in consumption of laboratory chow do not account for the changes in total caloric intake by the nicotine groups. In contrast, Fig. 3.3 reveals that the changes in caloric intake from the sugar solutions account for the changes in total caloric intake both during and after nicotine administration. The changes in caloric intake from the sugar solutions were significantly different between the nicotine and control groups. Therefore, the changes in caloric intake resulted from changes in consumption of specific foods rather than from changes in general food consumption.

An analysis of consumption of the three different sugar solutions available to the animals supports the conclusion that the changes in eating behavior resulted

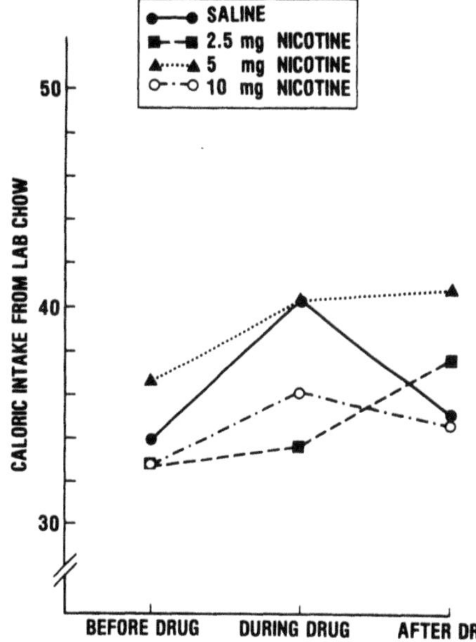

FIG. 3.2. Average caloric intake from laboratory chow before, during, and after drug administration. Reprinted with permission from Grunberg, 1982a *Addictive Behaviors*, 7, The effects of nicotine and cigarette smoking on food consumption and taste preferences, 1982, Pergamon Press, Ltd.

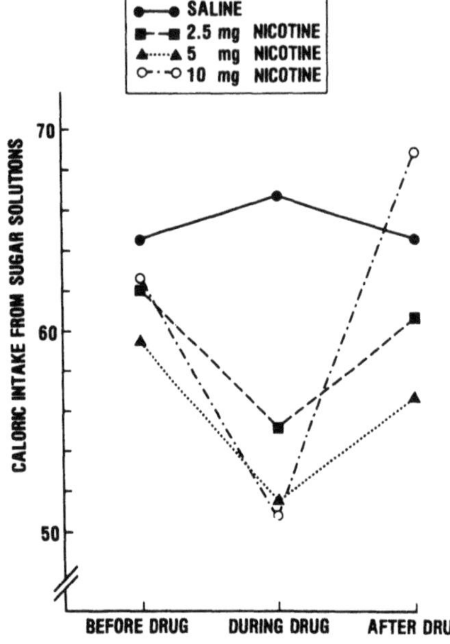

FIG. 3.3. Average caloric intake from sugar solutions before, during, and after drug administration. Reprinted with permission from Grunberg, 1982a *Addictive Behaviors*, 7, The effects of nicotine and cigarette smoking on food consumption and taste preferences, 1982, Pergamon Press, Ltd.

from changes in taste preferences (and specific food consumption). The control group consumed the same amounts of each of the three solutions throughout the experiment. In contrast, the nicotine groups decreased consumption of the two sweetest sugar solutions during nicotine administration and increased consumption of these solutions after nicotine administration.

This study demonstrated that nicotine affects body weight. In addition, changes in consumption of specific foods resulted in changes in caloric intake that paralleled the body weight changes. In order to examine the relationship between cigarette smoking and food consumption in humans, another study was conducted.

The human study was designed to determine whether cigarette smoking and abstinence from smoking affects general or specific food consumption. The subjects were 24 men and 18 women between 18 and 36 years old. Of these people, 28 (16 men and 12 women) smoked at least 15 cigarettes per day for at least two years. The other people (8 men and 6 women) were nonsmokers.

The smokers were divided into two different experimental groups: Smokers who were allowed to smoke before the study, and smokers who were not. All subjects were asked to taste nine different foods and to rate each food on a set of taste judgment scales. There were three sweet foods (chocolate, coffee cake, gumdrops), three salty foods (salami, salted peanuts, pretzels) and three bland foods (cheese, unsalted crackers, and unsalted peanuts). The study was cast within the context of a taste judgment study to insure that each subject tasted every food. It was emphasized to the subjects that they could eat as much or as little as they liked of each food while making their taste judgments and after they were finished rating the foods. After the tasting session, subjects were asked to pick three foods which they would eat in another part of the study. The bowls of food were weighed and recorded before and after the taste session. Subjects' choices of three foods also were recorded.

Fig. 3.4 presents the average amounts eaten of the sweet, salty, and bland foods by the three experimental groups. The smokers who were allowed to smoke ate significantly less sweets than did the nonsmokers ($p < 0.01$) and less sweets than did the smokers who were not allowed to smoke ($p < 0.10$). There were no differences among the groups in consumption of the salty or bland foods.

The selection of foods to eat later showed the same pattern. Nonsmokers expressed a significantly greater preference for sweet foods than did smokers who were allowed to smoke ($p = 0.05$, Fischer Exact Test). Smokers not

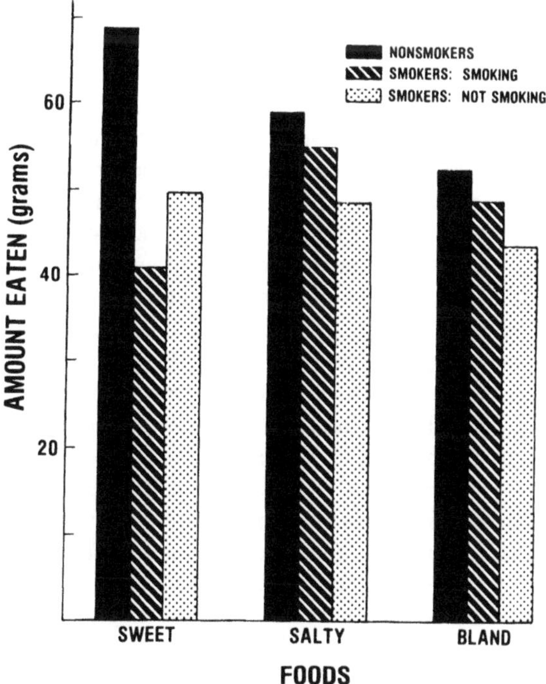

FIG. 3.4. Average amount of food eaten within each taste class. Reprinted with permission from Grunberg, 1982a *Addictive Behaviors*, 7, The effects of nicotine and cigarette smoking on food consumption and taste preferences, 1982, Pergamon Press, Ltd.

allowed to smoke also expressed a greater preference for sweet food compared to the smokers allowed to smoke ($p = 0.11$, Fischer Exact Test). The food preference of nonsmokers and smokers not allowed to smoke did not differ.

In both the human and animal studies, nicotine administration (or cigarette smoking) was accompanied by decreased consumption of specific foods; consumption of sweet foods decreased but consumption of nonsweet foods did not change. Abstinence from nicotine (or cigarette smoking) was accompanied by increased consumption of these specific foods. The animal study indicated that these changes in specific food consumption resulted in changes in caloric intake that paralleled changes in body weight. Therefore, the changes in caloric intake resulting from changes in specific food consumption contributed to the body weight changes. Because consumption of only specific foods changed, the relationship between nicotine and body weight could not be attributed to changes in general food consumption or general appetite. Instead, the eating changes in both studies were restricted to certain foods. The fact that the effect in humans was observed with sweet-tasting solid foods and that the effect in animals was observed with sweet-tasting liquids adds power to the conclusion that specific taste preferences were the key to the eating changes.

Based on these studies alone, there is a troublesome possibility that the results are limited to short-term laboratory settings. Before it can even be suggested that changes in taste preferences and specific food consumption could account for weight changes such as those observed in cancer cachexia, there must be some evidence that changes in specific food consumption occur outside the laboratory. A study by Grunberg and Morse (1984) is relevant to this point.

This study was designed to determine whether the results of the animal and human laboratory studies are generalizable on an epidemiological level to the United States population as a whole. United States per capita consumption of cigarettes was compared to United States per capita consumption of all major food groups for the years 1964 through 1977. These years were used because there was a marked decrease in U.S. cigarette consumption from 1969 through 1972 (during the Federal Government's intensive and highly publicized anti-smoking campaign) and because all of the required data are available only from 1964 through 1977. Correlations were computed between the per capita consumption of cigarettes and each major foodstuff on a yearly basis (41 comparisons were made). This study found substantial inverse correlations between U.S. per capita cigarette consumption and consumption of only a few specific foods. The inverse relationship between sugar and cigarette consumption was particularly striking. In fact, the partial correlation between cigarette and sugar consumption (holding sugar price constant) was statistically significant ($p < 0.05$). This study supports the conclusion of the laboratory study that cigarette smoking or nicotine administration alters specific food consumption and not general food consumption.

Taken together, this series of studies indicates that nicotine and cigarette smoking affect specific food consumption and taste preferences. The animal study demonstrates that this effect contributes to body weight changes. Based on this research and the clinical observations cited earlier, it seems reasonable to postulate that changes in specific food consumption and taste preferences may contribute to the weight changes in cancer cachexia.

CANCER CACHEXIA: CONSIDERATIONS FOR TREATMENTS AND RESEARCH

The fact that specific food consumption and taste preferences contributed to body weight changes in the nicotine studies indicates that this aspect of eating behavior can play a role in altering body weight. Considering this demonstration with the cancer literature cited earlier in this chapter, it may prove quite valuable to carefully examine taste preferences and specific food consumption in cancer patients. The existence of altered taste preferences certainly does not exclude learned taste aversions, learned taste preferences, or changes in taste acuity. Each of these phenomena may appear, and each must be examined and distinguished in order to understand the mechanisms of cancer cachexia and to design the most effective treatments.

Strategies of feeding and providing supplemental nutrients to cancer patients should consider and use eating changes to their advantage. For example, patients could be given a tray of actual foods to taste in order to choose their meals. The idea of a food preference tray has been suggested and used already by some oncologists and nutritionists (e.g., DeWys, 1980; DeWys & Herbst, 1977; Gormican, 1980; Holland, Rowland, & Plumb, 1977). Direct assessment of specific food preference avoids the problems raised earlier of extrapolating from eating studies that do not measure food consumption (e.g., taste acuity data)—problems such as threshold versus suprathreshold sensitivity, ratings of solids versus liquids, and judgments before or after eating. Each patient's food preferences should be determined directly and should use actual foods. This approach could be useful in both research evaluation of eating and in clinical treatment.

The food choice tray could easily be extended to determine what specific tastes or taste additives are most palatable. In addition, a food choice tray could be used to determine whether specific nutrients, vitamins, or food groups (e.g., carbohydrates versus fats versus proteins) are particularly liked or disliked. This simple approach could yield valuable new data while helping cancer patients maintain their body weight by providing preferred foods or by treating foods and nutrient supplements with preferred tastes. Also, nutrients and vitamins could be added to preferred foods.

Food preference choices should be reevaluated frequently to allow for cancer-related changes in taste preferences (such as phase of tumor growth and cancer treatment) and noncancer specific factors (such as nutritive state). In addition, once food preferences (and aversions) have been determined, this information might be put to optimal use by applying traditional behavioral modification techniques to control eating (cf. Grunberg, 1982b). For example, favorite tastes could be offered as rewards to encourage patients to eat other necessary nutrients that taste less pleasurable (and which cannot be adequately flavored). Quantities and frequency of meals also could be adjusted and doctored with preferred tastes to increase caloric intake.

Another possibility for increasing food consumption by cancer patients relies on the fact that the taste of foods may be altered with other foods and chemicals. For instance, consumption of miracle fruit (*Synsepalum dulcificum*) makes sour foods taste sweet. In contrast, chewing *Gymnema sylvestre* leaves suppresses the sweetness of sucrose and other foods (Bartoshuk, Dateo, Vandenbelt, Buttrick, & Long, 1969). In addition, exposure of the tongue to an artichoke makes water and other solutions taste sweet. It is important to recognize that this phenomenon does not result from providing a sweet-tasting substance. Instead, the tongue is temporarily altered and, as a result, a nonsweet substance tastes sweet (Bartoshuk, Lee, & Scarpellino, 1972). These types of effects suggest interesting possibilities for cancer patients. Once specific food and taste preferences are determined for a particular patient, caloric intake might be increased by altering food tastes in ways that follow from the empirical work of Bartoshuk and others. This possibility for altering taste and palatability of food to cancer patients deserves more research and clinical attention.

Another unexplored possibility is that caloric intake in cancer patients is affected by psychological (mental) states acting through physiological mechanisms. As an example, Schmale (1979) speculates that feelings of hopelessness may affect taste thresholds and caloric intake. (This possibility is quite different from a psychological state, such as depression, resulting in decreased food consumption because the patient has given up.) This suggestion raises the intriguing possibility that other psychological states may affect caloric intake by altering taste preferences, learned taste aversions, taste thresholds, or hunger; or that psychological states may affect caloric expenditure. For example, the psychological phenomenon of "perceived control" may be relevant to the issue of cancer cachexia because cancer patients generally cannot control their condition. A classic series of studies in experimental psychology by Glass and Singer (1972) investigated the effects of noise on people who could not turn off the noise and on people who believed they could terminate the noise. Subjects who had no control over the noise displayed deficits in behavioral and cognitive tasks after the noise had been discontinued. In contrast, subjects who believed that they could stop the noise ("perceived control"), but who were exposed to the same amount of noise as were subjects who could not control the noise, showed no deficits in performance afterwards. This effect also was demonstrated with other stressors (e.g., the annoyance of bureaucratic red tape). Although associations among perceived control of stressful states (e.g., an illness such as cancer), physiological changes, and behavior are somewhat speculative at this time, there is an increasing amount of empirical evidence that these types of relationships exist and may be substantial (see Baum, Grunberg, & Singer, 1982 for a discussion of psychological, behavioral, psychophysiological, and biochemical responses to stress). Investigators and clinicians should be alert to and consider these types of possibilities.

INCREASED BODY WEIGHT IN CANCER PATIENTS

This chapter began by describing a stereotyped cancer patient as thin and weak. However, oncologists and oncology nurses commonly find that breast cancer patients receiving chemotherapy gain substantial amounts of weight (e.g., at least 10–30 pounds) (DeConti, 1982; Knobf, Mullen, Xistris, & Moritz, 1983; M. Lippman, T. D'Angelo, & C. Gorrell, personal communication, 1982). Because this observation has not been carefully studied, it is not known whether the weight gains are a result of the tumor, the therapy, the patient's reaction to the cancer, or a combination of these possibilities. In addition, the relative contribution of psychological and physiological factors has not been established. If eating changes occur in these patients, it is unlikely that learned taste aversions are involved. Changes in taste preferences, specific food consumption, and general food consumption must be directly examined.

It remains possible that increases in body weight occur in other cancer patients as well. Body weight data must be systematically recorded and reported along with type of tumor, stage of tumor, and specific treatment. In addition, whether changes in body weight are increases or decreases, eating behavior must be carefully examined to determine what factors contribute to the weight changes. Only then can we develop effective treatments for the weight changes.

SUMMARY

Many cancer patients lose substantial amounts of weight and are malnourished. This condition is known as cachexia. The weight loss results from both psychological and physiological causes. The psychological causes mainly affect caloric intake. It has been suggested that the decreased caloric intake by cancer patients may result from learned taste aversions or changes in taste acuity. This chapter argues that changes in specific food consumption and taste preferences provide an alternative explanation that should be considered and examined. Clinical examples of changed taste preferences in cancer patients are cited. Data are presented from a recent series of studies demonstrating that changes in specific food consumption contribute to the changes in body weight associated with nicotine and cigarette smoking. Implications for treatment and research are suggested. Finally, it is noted that some cancer patients gain weight. Weight gains could not be explained by learned taste aversions. Body weight and eating behavior of cancer patients must be examined carefully and directly in order to understand the mechanisms involved in body weight changes and to develop the most effective ways to control these changes.

REFERENCES

Aker, S. N. (1979). Oral feedings in the cancer patient. *Cancer, 43,* 2103–2107.

Bartoshuk, L. M. (1978). The psychophysics of taste. *American Journal of Clinical Nutrition, 31,* 1068–1077.

Bartoshuk, L. M., Lee, C., & Scarpellino, R. (1972). Sweet taste of water induced by artichoke (cynara scolymus). *Science, 178,* 988–990.

Bartoshuk, L. M., Dateo, G. P., Vandenbelt, D. J., Buttrick, R. L., & Long, L., Jr. (1969). Effects of *Gymnema Sylvestre* and *Synsepalum dulcificum* on taste in man. In C. Pfaffman (Ed.), *Olfaction and taste. III.* New York: Rockfeller University Press.

Baum, A., Grunberg, N. E., & Singer, J. E. (1982). The use of psychological and neuroendocrinological measurements in the study of stress. *Health Psychology, 1,* 217–236.

Bernstein, I. L. (1978). Learned taste aversions in children receiving chemotherapy. *Science, 200,* 1302–1303.

Bernstein, I. L., & Bernstein, I. D. (1981). Learned food aversions and cancer anorexia. *Cancer Treatment Reports, 65,* (Suppl. 5), 43–47.

Bernstein, I. L., & Sigmundi, R. A. (1980). Tumor anorexia: A learned food aversion? *Science, 209,* 416–418.

Bernstein, I. L., Vitiello, M. V., & Sigmundi, R. A. (1980). Effects of tumor growth on taste-aversion learning produced by antitumor drugs in the rat. *Physiological Psychology, 8,* 51–55.

Bernstein, I. L., Wallace, M. J., Bernstein, I. D., Bleyer, W. A., Chard, R. L., & Hartmann, J. R. (1979). Learned food aversions as a consequence of cancer treatment. In J. van Eys, M. S. Seelig, & B. L. Nichols (Eds.), *Nutrition and cancer.* New York: S. P. Medical and Scientific Books.

Birch, D. (1975). Control: Cigarettes and calories. *Canadian Nurse, 71,* 33–35.

Bolles, R. C., Hayward, L., & Crandall, C. (1981). Conditioned taste preferences based on caloric density. *Journal of Experimental Psychology: Animal Behavior Processes, 7,* 59–69.

Brewin, T. B. (1980). Can a tumor cause the same appetite perversion or taste change as a pregnancy? *Lancet, 2,* (8200), 907–908.

Briese, E. & Quijada, M. (1979). Positive alliesthesia after insulin. *Experientia, 35,* 1058–1059.

Buzby, G. P., & Steinberg, J. J. (1981). Nutrition in cancer patients. *Surgical Clinics of North America, 61,* 691–700.

Cabanac, M. (1971). Physiological role of pleasure. *Science, 173,* 1103–1107.

Cabanac, M., Minaire, Y., & Adair, E. R. (1968). Influence of internal factors on the pleasantness of a gustative sweet sensation. *Communications in Behavioral Biology,* Part A, *1,* 77–82.

Capaldi, E. D., & Myers, D. E. (1982). Taste preferences as a function of food deprivation during original taste exposure. *Animal Learning & Behavior, 10,* 211–219.

Carson, J. A. S., & Gormican, A. (1977). Taste activity & food attitudes of selected patients with cancer. *Journal of the American Dietetic Association, 70,* 361–365.

Chlebowski, R. T., Heber, D., & Block, J. B. (1981). Metabolic evaluation prior to and following development of cachexia in lung cancer patients. (Abstr.) *Proceedings of the American Association for Cancer Research, 22,* 424.

Comroe, J. H., Jr. (1960). The pharmacological actions of nicotine. *Annals of the New York Academy of Sciences, 90,* 48–51.

Costa, G. (1963). Cachexia, the metabolic component of neoplastic diseases. *Progress in Experimental Tumor Research, 3,* 321–369.

Costa, G., & Donaldson, S. S. (1979). Effects of cancer and cancer treatment on the nutrition of the host. *New England Journal of Medicine, 300,* 1471–1474.

Davidson-Codjoe, M., & Holman, E. W. (1982). The effect of nonnutritive satiation on the learning of a flavor preference by rats. *Animal Learning & Behavior, 10,* 220–222.

DeConti, R. C. (1982). Weight gain in the adjuvant chemotherapy of breast cancer. *American Society of Clinical Oncology Abstracts,* C-279, 73.

DeWys, W. D. (1974). Abnormalities of taste as a remote effect of a neoplasm. *Annals New York Academy of Sciences, 230,* 427–434.

DeWys, W. D. (1977). Changes in taste sensation in cancer patients: Correlation with caloric intake. In M. R. Kare & O. Maller (Eds.), *The chemical senses and nutrition.* New York: Academic Press.

DeWys, W. D. (1978). Changes in taste sensation and feeding behavior in cancer patients: A review. *Journal of Human Nutrition, 32,* 447–453.

DeWys, W. D. (1979). Anorexia as a general effect of cancer. *Cancer, 43,* 2013–2019.

DeWys, W. D. (1980). Nutritional care of the cancer patient. *Journal of the American Medical Association, 244,* 374–376.

DeWys, W. D., Costa, G., & Henkin, R. (1981). Clinical parameters related to anorexia. *Cancer Treatment Reports, 65* (Suppl. 5), 49–52.

DeWys, W. D., & Herbst, S. H. (1977). Oral feeding in the nutritional management of the cancer patient. *Cancer Research, 37,* 2429–2431.

DeWys, W. D., & Walters, K. (1975). Abnormalities of taste sensation in cancer patients. *Cancer, 36,* 1888–1896.

Donaldson, S. S. (1977). Nutritional consequences of radiotherapy. *Cancer Research, 37,* 2407–2413.

Donaldson, S. S., & Lenon, R. A. (1979). Alterations of nutritional status: Impact of chemotherapy and radiation therapy. *Cancer, 43,* 2036–2052.

Dudgeon, B. J., DeLisa, J. A., & Miller, R. M. (1980). Head and neck cancer, a rehabilitation approach. *American Journal of Occupational Therapy, 34,* 243–251.

Garattini, S., Bizzi, A., Donelli, M. G., Guaitani, A., Samanin, R., & Spreafico, F. (1980). Anorexia and cancer in animals and man. *Cancer Treatment Reviews, 7,* 115–140.

Garcia, J., Hankins, W. G., & Rusiniak, K. W. (1974). Behavioral regulation of the milieu interne in man and rat. *Science, 185,* 824–831.

Garcia, J., Kimeldorf, D. J., & Koelling, R. A. (1955). Conditioned aversion to saccharin resulting from exposure to gamma radiation. *Science, 122,* 157–158.

Garcia, J., & Koelling, R. A. (1967). A comparison of aversions induced by X-rays, toxins, and drugs in the rat. *Radiation Research Supplement, 7,* 439–450.

Glass, D. C., & Singer, J. E. (1972). *Urban Stress.* New York: Academic Press.

Gormican, A. (1980). Influencing food acceptance in anorexic cancer patients. *Postgraduate Medicine, 68,* 145–7, 150–2.

Gorshein, D. (1977). Posthypophysectomy taste abnormalities—their relationship to remote effects of cancer. *Cancer, 39,* 1700–1703.

Grunberg, N. E. (1982a). The effects of nicotine and cigarette smoking on food consumption and taste preferences. *Addictive Behaviors, 7,* 317–331.

Grunberg, N. E. (1982b). Obesity: Etiology, hazards, and treatment. In R. J. Gatchel, A. Baum, &

J. E. Singer (Eds.), *Handbook of psychology and health, Vol. 1.* Hillsdale, N.J: Lawrence Erlbaum Associates.

Grunberg, N. E., & Morse, D. E. (1984). Cigarette smoking and food consumption in the United States. *Journal of Applied Social Psychology, 14.*

Hall, J. C. (1979). The cachexia of cancer. *Biomedicine, 30,* 287–291.

Henkin, R. I., Gill, J. R., & Bartter, F. C. (1963). Studies of taste thresholds in normal man and in patients with adrenal cortical insufficiency: The role of adrenal cortical steroids and of serum sodium concentration. *Journal of Clinical Investigation, 42,* 727–735.

Holland, J. C. B., Rowland, J., & Plumb, M. (1977). Psychological aspects of anorexia in cancer patients. *Cancer Research, 37,* 2425–2428.

Kaplan, A. R., & Powell, W. (1969). Taste acuity in relation to hunger. *Nature, 221,* 367–368.

Knobf, M. K., Mullen, J. C., Xistris, D., & Moritz, D. A. (1983). Weight gain in women with breast cancer receiving adjuvant chemotherapy. *Oncology Nursing Forum, 10,* 28–33.

Mackey, A. O., & Jones, P. (1954). Selection of members of a food tasting panel: Discernment of primary tastes in water solution compared with judging ability for foods. *Food Technology, 8,* 527–530.

Morrison, S. D. (1976). Control of food intake in cancer cachexia: A challenge and a tool. *Physiology and Behavior, 17,* 705–714.

Morrison, S. D. (1978). Origins of anorexia in neoplastic disease. *American Journal of Clinical Nutrition, 31,* 1104–1107.

Morrison, S. D. (1979). Anorexia and the cancer patient. In J. van Eys, M. S. Seelig, & B. L. Nichols (Eds.), *Nutrition and cancer.* New York: S. P. Medical and Scientific Books.

Moskowitz, H. R., Kumraiah, V., Sharma, K. N., Jacobs, H., & Sharma, S. D. (1976). Effects of hunger, satiety and glucose load upon taste intensity and taste hedonics. *Physiology and Behavior, 16,* 471–475.

Mossman, K. L., & Henkin, R. I. (1978). Radiation-induced changes in taste acuity in cancer patients. *International Journal of Radiation Oncology, Biology, Physics, 4,* 663–670.

Myrsten, A., Elgerot, A., & Edgren, B. (1977). Effects of abstinence from tobacco smoking on physiological and psychological arousal levels in habitual smokers. *Psychosomatic Medicine, 39,* 25–38.

Nielsen, S. S., Theologides, A., & Vickers, Z. M. (1980). Influence of food odors on food aversions and preferences in patients with cancer. *American Journal of Clinical Nutrition, 33,* 2253–2261.

Ohnuma, T., & Holland, J. (1977). Nutritional consequences of cancer chemotherapy and immunotherapy. *Cancer Research, 37,* 2395–2406.

Pangborn, R. M., & Trabue, I. M. (1967). Detection and apparent taste intensity of salt-acid mixtures in two media. *Perception and Psychophysics, 2,* 503–509.

Passey, R. D., Elson, L. A., & Connors, T. A. (1961). Growth and metabolic effects of cigarette smoking and nicotine inhalation. *British Empire Cancer Campaign Annual Report, 39,* Part II, 90.

Rose, J. C. (1978). Nutritional problems in radiotherapy patients. *American Journal of Nursing, 78,* 1194–1196.

Rozin, P., & Kalat, J. W. (1971). Specific hungers and poison avoidance as adaptive specializations of learning. *Psychological Review, 78,* 459–486.

Russ, J. E., & DeWys, W. D. (1978). Correction of taste abnormality of malignancy with intravenous hyperalimentation. *Archives of Internal Medicine, 138,* 799–800.

Russell, M. A. H. (1971). Cigarette smoking: Natural history of a dependence disorder. *The British Journal of Medical Psychology, 28,* 418.

Schachter, S. (1978). Pharmacological and psychological determinants of smoking. *Annals of Internal Medicine, 88,* 104–114.

Schechter, M. D., & Cook, P. G. (1976). Nicotine-induced weight loss in rats without an effect on appetite. *European Journal of Pharmacology, 38,* 63–69.

Schein, P. S., Macdonald, J. S., Waters, C., & Haidak, D. (1975). Nutritional complications of cancer and its treatment. *Seminars in Oncology, 2,* 337–347.

Schmale, A. H. (1979). Psychological aspects of anorexia: Areas for study. *Cancer, 43,* 2087–2092.

Settle, R. G., Quinn, M. R., Brand, J. G., Kare, M. R., Mullen, J. L., & Brown, R. (1979). Gustatory evaluation of cancer patients: Preliminary results. In J. van Eys, M. S. Seelig, & B. L. Nichols (Eds.), *Nutrition and cancer.* New York: S. P. Medical and Scientific Books.

Shils, M. E. (1979). Nutricial problems induced by cancer. *Medical Clinics of North America, 63,* 1009–1025.

Smith, J. C., & Blumsack, J. T. (1981). Learned taste aversion as a factor in cancer therapy. *Cancer Treatment Reports, 65,* (Suppl. 5), 37–42.

Theologides, A. (1977). Nutritional management of the patient with advanced cancer *Postgraduate Medicine, 61,* 97–101.

Theeuwes, F., & Yum, S. I. (1977). Principles of the design and operation of generic osmotic pumps for the delivery of semisolid or liquid drug formulations. *Annals of Biomedical Engineering, 4,* 343–353.

Thompson, D. A., & Campbell, R. G. (1977). Hunger in humans induced by 2-deoxy-D-glucose: Glucoprivic control of taste preference and food intake. *Science, 198,* 1065–1068.

Trant, A. S., Serin, J., & Douglass, H. O. (1982). Is taste related to anorexia in cancer patients? *American Journal of Clinical Nutrition, 36,* 45–58.

Wack, J. T., & Rodin, J. (1982). Smoking and its effects on body weight and the systems of caloric regulation. *The American Journal of Clinical Nutrition, 35,* 366–380.

Waterhouse, C. (1963). Nutritional disorders in neoplastic disease. *Journal of Chronic Diseases, 16,* 637–644.

Williams, L. R., & Cohen, M. H. (1978). Altered taste thresholds in lung cancer. *American Journal of Clinical Nutrition, 31,* 122–125.

Young, V. R. (1977). Energy metabolism and requirements in the cancer patient. *Cancer Research, 37,* 2336–2347.

Zahorik, D. M. (1977). Associative and non-associative factors in learned food preferences. In L. M. Barker, M. R. Best, & M. Domjan (Eds.), *Learning Mechanisms in Food Selection.* Waco TX: Baylor University Press.

II TASTE AVERSIONS AND EATING BEHAVIOR IN CANCER

4 Learned Food Aversions and Tumor Anorexia

Ilene L. Bernstein
Charles M. Treneer
University of Washington

Roughly two-thirds of all patients who die of cancer display anorexia and weight loss prior to death (Morrison, 1976). Therapeutic interventions and physical obstructions created by the growth and spread of neoplastic tissue are sometimes responsible for reductions in food intake (Costa & Donaldson, 1979; Ohnuma & Holland, 1977; Schein, Macdonald, Waters, & Haidak, 1974). However, a number of clinical and experimental tumors are associated with hypophagia and weight loss in the absence of aversive therapy or gastrointestinal obstruction. The physiological bases of this hypophagia remain unclear. Some researchers have speculated that tumor growth may be associated with elevations in brain serotonin (Krause, James, Ziparo & Fischer, 1979) or circulating peptides (Mordes & Rossini, 1981) which act directly to produce suppression of appetite. Although we agree that "direct" effects of tumor growth may well play an important role in tumor-induced anorexia, we have proposed that tumor growth may also suppress appetite indirectly by producing chronic symptoms which act as unconditioned stimuli (USs) in the acquisition of learned food aversions.

This chapter reviews our original research implicating a role for learned food aversions in tumor anorexia and describes some of the recent directions this work has taken. We are currently seeking answers to three major questions: (1) What is the overall contribution of learned food aversions to tumor anorexia? (2) How general are tumor-induced aversions? and (3) What are the physiological mechanisms responsible for the development of tumor-induced aversions?

LEARNED FOOD AVERSIONS ARE ASSOCIATED WITH TUMOR ANOREXIA

Garcia and his colleagues first reported that when animals ingest a particular food or liquid before receiving a drug or radiation treatment that induces gastrointestinal (GI) discomfort, they will subsequently reduce their intake of that substance or avoid ingesting it altogether (Garcia, Ervin, & Koelling, 1966; Garcia, Hankins, & Rusiniak, 1974). This phenomenon has been termed food or taste aversion learning and is usually described as a variant of classical conditioning in which animals learn to associate a conditioned stimulus (CS) (the taste) with an unconditioned stimulus (US) (the illness). Taste aversion learning has received a great deal of attention in recent years because it appears to be an unusually robust type of learning marked by extremely rapid acquisition and a high resistance to extinction. Learning theorists have suggested that food aversion learning enables animals to successfully avoid ingesting toxic substances and to select foods with needed nutrients (Bolles, 1975; Rozin & Kalat, 1971). We have suggested that similar symptoms could develop as a consequence of tumor growth or antitumor therapy and give rise to similar types of learning via the same associative mechanisms. In this case, however, the learning would have no particular adaptive value for the organism. Our earliest work indicated that learned food aversions occur in patients receiving drug treatments that cause severe and unpleasant side effects (Bernstein, 1978). We subsequently began to ask whether learned food aversions were of more general significance, that is, if aversions arose in response to the association of a diet with the aversive physiological effects of the tumor itself. We reasoned that tumor-induced appetite loss, like drug-induced appetite loss, could be based on learned aversions, with the US being some chronic symptom of tumor growth rather than the acute effects of a drug injection (Bernstein & Sigmundi, 1980).

To investigate this hypothesis, we implanted a transplantable, polyoma-virus induced sarcoma (PW-739) subcutaneously in the flanks of syngeneic Wistar-Furth rats. Control animals received an incision and suture but no tumors. The growth of this tumor is associated with significant depressions in food intake and body weight which typically begin approximately five to six weeks after the tumor is implanted. To determine whether a novel diet would become aversive by virtue of its presentation during the period of illness, tumor-bearing and control animals were exposed to a distinctive target diet (AIN meal,[1] ICN, Cleveland, Ohio) for ten days and then tested for the presence of aversions. At the end of the diet exposure period the food intake of tumor-bearing animals had declined significantly below that of controls. Aversions were assessed by offering the animals two diets (AIN and "chocolate chow"[2]) simultaneously for 24 hours and measuring their consumption of each. We calculated preference scores for each animal by dividing the amount of AIN diet consumed by total amount of

[1]AIN diet consists of casein (20%), corn starch (15%), sucrose (50%), fiber (5%), corn oil (5%), mineral mix (3.5%), vitamin mix (1%), choline bitartrate (0.2%), and DL-methionine (0.3%).

[2]Novel diet of comparable palatability to the AIN diet (in untreated animals) was composed of five parts ground Purina rat chow; five parts Carnation chocolate instant breakfast mix, and one part Crisco vegetable oil, by volume.

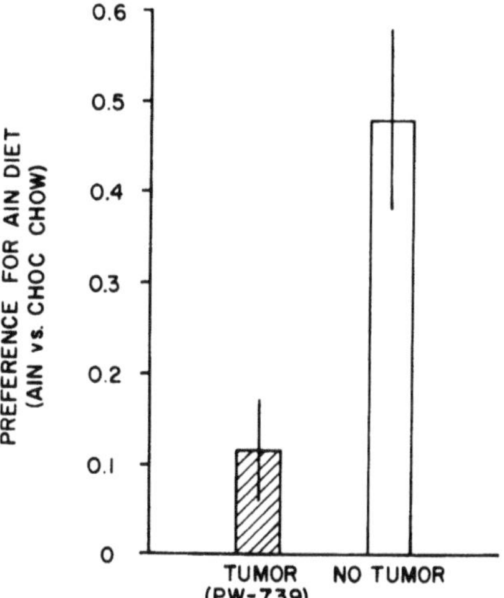

FIG. 4.1. Average preference [± standard error of the mean (S.E.M.)] for AIN meal in the 24-hour two-food choice test (AIN meal versus chocolate chow). Average total consumption: tumor, 18.3 g; control, 17.4 g. (Reprinted from Bernstein & Sigmundi, 1980 with permission: Copyright 1980 by the AAAS).

food consumed over the 24-hour test; low scores indicate low preference for the target (AIN) diet.

Mean AIN preference scores are depicted in Fig. 4.1. Tumor-bearing animals exhibited conspicuously lower preferences than controls for the AIN diet ($p < .01$; t test), the diet which had been available during recent tumor growth. Furthermore, when an alternate diet was available during the preference test, we saw striking elevations of 24-hr food intake (85% increase over pretest intake) in tumor-bearing animals but not in controls. These findings indicate that the tumor-bearing animals had developed a pronounced aversion to the AIN target diet by the day of the preference test.

In additional studies, aversions were shown to be specific to the particular diet available during tumor growth, thus excluding the possibility that our original findings were a nonspecific effect of tumor growth on taste preference. We have concluded that tumor-induced aversions are based on learning, that is, the association of a specific food with some symptom(s) of tumor growth.

ASSESSING THE CONTRIBUTION OF LEARNED FOOD AVERSIONS TO ANOREXIA

Because there is clear evidence that learned food aversions arise in tumor-bearing animals, an important question is whether the preference shifts which characterize "learned aversions" can actually lead to hypophagia and significant weight loss. It is important to distinguish between depressions in food intake which are the direct result of tumor-induced physiological changes and those which are truly the consequence of learned aversions. We chose to begin our investigations by modeling the effects of a tumor in undiseased animals (Bernstein & Goehler, 1983). We used osmotic minipumps (Alza, Palo Alto, Calif.), which are small, implantable capsules, to provide a continuous infusion of a concentrated solution of lithium chloride (LiCl) over a seven day period. They provide a controlled chemical simulation of the kind of chronic US exposure experienced by tumor-bearing animals. To separate learned from direct effects, we compared the response to LiCl infusions of animals consuming their familiar maintenance diet to those consuming a novel diet. Familiar tastes are relatively resistant to the development of learned food aversions whereas novel tastes rapidly become the target of such aversions (Revusky & Bedarf, 1967). Thus, even though drug infusions were the same in both groups, the likelihood of forming strong aversions was quite different since the group with a novel diet had a more salient target. Differences in food intake would be a reflection of greater learned aversions in the novel food group.

One day prior to implantation of the minipumps, we assigned weight-matched Wistar rats to either Novel diet groups (which were given ad lib access to a novel diet (C-21[3]) in place of their usual diet) or Familiar diet groups (which received their usual Wayne Lab Blox in ground form). The next day, we implanted an osmotic minipump in the peritoneal cavity of each subject. We gave half the animals in each diet condition (Drug-Novel and Drug-Familiar groups) minipumps containing 300 μl of a saturated aqueous solution of LiCl. The pumps deliver a relatively constant ip infusion of solution (one μl per hour) for approximately eight days. Control animals (Control-Novel and Control-Familiar groups) received nonfunctional pumps. After implantation animals continued to have free access to their assigned diet for six days. On Day 7 we tested for the presence of aversions in a 24-hour two food preference test. The two foods provided in the test were the target diet, (either ground Wayne chow for familiar diet groups or C-21 for novel diet groups) and AIN meal (a diet novel to both groups). Preference scores for the target diet were determined for individual animals by dividing the amount of target diet consumed by the total food consumed during the preference test.

Following the preference test we switched half the animals in each group to the AIN while allowing the remaining animals to continue on the same diets they had consumed during the infusion period. In this manner we determined whether the availability of a new, nonaversive diet at the time the animals were recovering from the effects of drug infusions would be associated with more rapid increases in food intake.

Daily food intake during drug infusion is presented in Fig. 4.2. Striking differences in food intake between Novel and Familiar drug treated animals are apparent; chronic drug infusions produced significantly more anorexia in animals

[3]C-21 diet consists of casein (20%), sucrose (15%), corn starch (35.4%), Crisco shortening (24%), salt mixture (4%), codliver oil (1%), choline chloride (0.1%), DL-methionine (0.5%), plus vitamin mix.

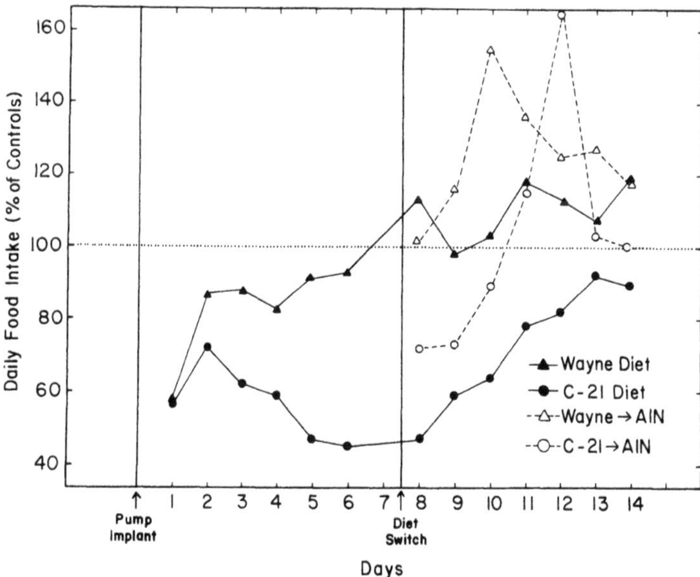

FIG. 4.2. Mean daily food intake of animals receiving chronic LiCl infusion, expressed as percentage of intake of control animals on the same diet. (Wayne diet was familiar; C-21 was novel.) Mean daily control intakes during the infusion period were 13.8 g on Wayne and 11.8 g on C-21. (Reprinted with permission from Bernstein & Goehler, 1983. Copyright 1983 by the American Psychological Association).

consuming a novel food than in those consuming familiar, Wayne chow. Furthermore, significant food aversions developed in animals with a novel diet–drug association (*t* test; $p < .05$) but not in animals with a familiar diet–drug association ($p > .1$).

Two factors were likely to contribute to the decline of food intake associated with minipump infusions. One factor is the direct or unconditioned effect of drug-induced malaise on appetite. Such discomfort would presumably afflict novel and familiar groups equally. The other factor is the conditioned effect and results from food aversions which arise due to diet–illness associations. As expected, the novel diet proved much more susceptible to these conditioned effects. The development of diet aversions in the novel but not the familiar diet group enabled us to assess the potential contribution of learned aversions to the anorexia produced by a chronic, aversive US. The considerable difference in appetite suppression in animals on familiar and novel diets, we would argue, is largely attributable to learned food aversions. Support for the hypothesis that aversions can lead to anorexia was also provided by the effects on food intake of switching diets. Animals maintained on the same diet during the infusion and postinfusion period ate considerably less during the latter period than the animals switched to a new diet for the post-infusion period. Differences between the "switched" groups and the "same" groups were not due to lingering effects of the US (which were not different) but to the degree to which learned aversions were likely to affect intake.

A second study confirmed that it was novelty of the C-21 diet and not intrinsic differences between C-21 and Wayne lab chow which was responsible for differences in intake suppression. In this study, novel and familiar groups consumed the same diet (C-21) during the infusion period but differed in their prior experience with it. Significant anorexia appeared in animals unfamiliar with the diet but not in those familiar with it, which supports the hypothesis that differential intakes were due not to nutritional or taste properties of the diets but to novelty and differential aversion conditioning.

The striking effects of diet novelty on food intake in the previous study led us to examine whether parallel effects would be found in tumor-bearing animals. Similar findings would provide strong evidence of a major role for learned aversions in tumor anorexia. Specifically, the hypothesis that tumors suppress appetite directly would not predict a differential effect of diet novelty on severity of appetite depression, whereas the hypothesis that learned aversions contribute substantially to tumor-induced anorexia would predict less depression in animals eating a familiar diet than in those eating a novel diet. When we compared the food intake and preferences of tumor-bearing rats consuming a novel diet to those of rats consuming a familiar diet, we found that animals which consumed the familiar maintenance diet (Wayne lab chow) did not develop aversions to it and had relatively mild transient anorexia. In contrast, tumor-bearing animals consuming a novel diet (C-21) developed strong aversions to that diet and displayed severe anorexia (Bernstein, Treneer, Goehler & Murochick, submitted). These results are consistent with the hypothesis that differential food aversion conditioning can lead to the striking differences in severity of anorexia in tumor-bearing animals consuming "familiar" and "novel" diets.

Although animals consuming the familiar diet did not develop learned aversions, they did manifest anorexia and body weight deficits relative to healthy controls. This clearly indicates that factors other than learned aversions can lead to anorexia in animals with PW-739 tumors. Thus, we would not argue that learned food aversions are the only cause of tumor anorexia. However, the considerable differences seen between novel and familiar diet groups suggest strongly that learned food aversions can make a substantial contribution to anorexia in tumor-bearing animals.

ASSESSING THE GENERALITY OF TUMOR-INDUCED AVERSIONS

Other experimental tumors besides the PW-739 have been used in recent years to study the physiological bases of tumor-induced anorexia. These include the

Walker 256 carcinosarcoma (Krause et al, 1979; Morrison, 1973) and a Leydig cell tumor (LTW[m]) (Mordes & Rossini, 1981). Although growth of all three transplantable tumors is associated with significant declines of food intake and body weight, the mechanisms responsible for this anorexia may be different. The Walker tumor is a rapidly growing tumor which constitutes a substantial portion (30%) of the animal's body weight at the time significant declines in food intake become apparent (Morrison, 1973; Morrison, 1976). The Leydig tumor, on the other hand, produces symptoms of appetite loss when the tumor itself weighs less than a gram (Mordes & Rossini, 1981). The PW-739 tumor is intermediate in its growth rate and effects on food intake and body weight. We were therefore interested in comparing the effects on food intake and diet preferences of the Walker and Leydig tumors to our observations with PW-739 tumors.

In separate studies patterned after our original work with PW-739 tumors (Bernstein & Fenner, 1983), animals were implanted with either Leydig or Walker tumors and exposed to AIN or C-21 as their target diets for three to four weeks. We measured food intake daily and administered a preference test after anorexia was evident. We observed significant declines in food intake in animals with Leydig tumors at 17 days post-implant and in animals with Walker tumors at four weeks post-implant. Results of the preference tests can be seen in Tables 4.1 and 4.2. Animals with Leydig tumors, like those with PW-739 tumors, developed strong aversions to the specific diet they had been eating after tumor implant. On the other hand, animals with Walker tumors did not develop diet aversions, but instead displayed preferences for target diet which were indistinguishable from those of healthy controls. In addition, animals with Leydig tumors displayed significant elevations in food intake during preference testing (when an alternate diet was available) while those with Walker tumors did not.

Although Walker and Leydig tumors were both associated with significant declines in food intake, their effects on target diet preference were different. Contrasting responses to the availability of an alternative diet, as well as differential appearance of diet aversions, support the idea that learned food aversions

TABLE 4.1

Preference Test Scores:[a] Walker 256 Tumors

Ain Target	
Tumor	0.01 (±.01)
Control	0.07 (±.03)
C-21 Target	
Tumor	0.81 (±.03)
Control	0.78 (±.03)

[a]Preference test scores = grams of target diet consumed divided by total food consumption during the test.

TABLE 4.2
Preference Test Scores:[a] Leydig-LTW (M) Tumors

Ain Target	
Tumor	0.13 (±.05)
Control	0.40 (±.08)
C-21 Target	
Tumor	0.14 (±.08)
Control	0.69 (±.07)

[a]Preference test scores = grams of target diet consumed divided by total food consumption during the test.

contribute to anorexia in animals with Leydig but not Walker tumors. These findings emphasize that there are multiple factors contributing to the decline in food intake accompanying tumor growth and that "tumor anorexia" is not a unitary phenomenon with a single cause. It is likely that the clinical picture is at least as heterogeneous.

ASSESSING THE PHYSIOLOGICAL BASIS OF TUMOR-INDUCED AVERSIONS

The presence of learned aversions in animals with certain tumors indicates that physiological consequences of tumor growth can act as USs in aversion conditioning. Since we have found that the induction of food aversions is not common to all experimental rat tumors, it appears that illness and tumor growth per se are not sufficient conditions for the development of aversions. This suggests that tumor-induced aversions are caused by specific physiological changes, not merely by general malaise, and that these changes may prove identifiable.

In considering potential candidates for the physiological USs responsible for tumor-induced aversions, two categories of stimuli come to mind. One is substances secreted abnormally or in unusually large amounts by the tumor. It is possible that some substances have toxic effects which can act as USs in food aversion conditioning. The other possibility is that tumor growth produces a state of nutrient deficiency in the host organism by virtue of its excessive and preferential access to some essential nutrient(s) (Lawson, Richmond, Nixon, & Rudman, 1982). Thus, tumor-bearing animals' striking similarity to animals on nutrient deficient diets (See Rozin & Kalat, 1971) may be more than coincidental. Although the diets used in our studies are nutritionally adequate for normal animals, the tumor-bearing animals may be experiencing a physiological nutrient deficiency because the tumor receives preferential access to essential nutrients.

The amino acids constitute one group of nutrients known to be influenced by tumor growth (Goodlad, 1964; Wu & Bauer, 1960). Imbalances and deficiencies in essential amino acids can produce both declines in food intake and abnormal plasma amino acid profiles (Harper, Benevenga, & Wohlhueter, 1970; Rogers & Leung, 1977). We have recently begun to investigate whether nutritional deficiencies, particularly amino acid imbalances or deficiencies, are responsible for tumor-induced food aversions and anorexia.

In our initial investigations, we determined whether PW-739 tumor growth is associated with the development of abnormalities in plasma amino acids. We matched tumor-bearing animals to controls on the basis of body weight and food intake for the purpose of pair-feeding. For three weeks, each control animal received the amount of food its matched tumor-bearing animal had eaten the previous day. We obtained blood samples after significant anorexia appeared and had full profile amino acid assays done on the plasma fractions. Of the essential amino acids, only tryptophan was significantly depressed. Concentrations of total tryptophan in the plasma of tumor-bearing animals were approximately half the levels seen in controls. In addition, a number of essential and nonessential amino acids were significantly elevated in the plasma of tumor bearers (e.g. lysine, glutamic acid, aspartic acid, glycine, taurine). Thus, amino acid profiles were consistent with the hypothesis that PW-739 tumor growth leads to a deficiency or imbalance of plasma tryptophan. An imbalance exists when low levels of one essential amino acid occur in conjunction with higher than normal levels of other amino acids. Since pair-fed controls were used, it is not likely that abnormalities in the amino acid profiles of tumor-bearing animals were secondary to low food intake. However, pair-fed animals are likely to consume their restricted ration soon after being fed; their actual intake patterns were probably different from those of freely-feeding animals. When we repeated the plasma tryptophan assay with animals fed ad lib, we still found depressed tryptophan levels in tumor-bearing animals relative to controls. This suggests that the differences we observed were not due to differences in the feeding patterns of pair-fed and freely-feeding animals.

We next examined the temporal relationship between tumor-induced declines in tryptophan and anorexia. We obtained plasma samples at weekly intervals after tumor implant and assayed them for tryptophan concentration. We observed a gradual decline in plasma tryptophan as tumor growth advanced. Significant differences between tryptophan levels in tumor-bearing and control animals were evident approximately two weeks before the appearance of significant differences in food intake. Thus, the temporal relationship between declining tryptophan and anorexia in these animals further suggests that tryptophan deficiency is not secondary to anorexia because it precedes it in time.

Since initial studies suggested that depressions in tryptophan occur in tumor-bearing animals, we created tryptophan deficiencies in normal rats (Treneer & Bernstein, 1981) to verify that tryptophan deficiency could lead to anorexia.

Healthy animals were maintained on a tryptophan-free target diet or the same diet supplemented with L-tryptophan (0.5% of the diet) for ten days in order to determine whether diet-induced plasma tryptophan deficiency produces a behavioral syndrome similar to PW-739 tumor growth—namely, declines in food intake and the development of diet aversions. Rats maintained on a tryptophan-free diet showed significant depressions of plasma tryptophan. They also consumed significantly less food than rats receiving the same diet supplemented with L-tryptophan. When given a choice between the target diet and a novel alternative, the deficient animals displayed significantly lower target diet preferences than controls. Thus, healthy animals fed a tryptophan-free diet are similar to PW-739 tumor-bearing animals in showing significant depressions in plasma tryptophan, food intake, and preference for their diet. These findings are consistent with the hypothesis that tumor-induced amino acid deficiencies—in this instance, tryptophan deficiencies—can contribute to anorexia and learned food aversions. If tryptophan deficiencies or imbalances contribute to tumor anorexia, it may be possible to restore normal tryptophan levels via dietary supplements and thereby prevent or postpone tumor-induced anorexia.

SUMMARY

The studies discussed in this chapter examined whether learned food aversions contribute to the anorexia which arises as a result of tumor growth. Tumor growth was found to be associated with the development of strong aversions to the available diet. Immediate elevations in food intake occurred when a new food was introduced. Thus, learned aversions to the specific diet eaten during tumor growth appear to play a causal role in the development of tumor-induced anorexia.

The food aversions apparent in animals with certain experimental tumors point to physiological consequences of tumor growth which act as unconditioned stimuli in taste aversion conditioning. Identification of the physiological changes responsible for these aversions could point the way to straightforward and effective clinical interventions for preventing aversions and alleviating symptoms of anorexia.

ACKNOWLEDGMENT

This research was supported by NIH grant RO1-CA26419.

REFERENCES

Bernstein, I. L. (1978). Learned taste aversions in children receiving chemotherapy. *Science, 200,* 1302–1303.

Bernstein, I. L., & Fenner, D. P. (1983). Learned food aversions: Heterogeneity of animal models of tumor-induced anorexia. *Appetite, 4,* 79–86.

Bernstein, I. L., & Goehler, L. E. (1983). Chronic lithium chloride infusions: Conditioned suppression of food intake and preference. *Behavioral Neuroscience, 97,* 290–298.

Bernstein, I. L., & Sigmundi, R. A. (1980). Tumor anorexia: A learned food aversion? *Science, 209,* 416–418.

Bernstein, I. L., Treneer, C. M., Goehler, L. E., & Murochick, E. (submitted). *Tumor growth in rats: Conditioned suppression of food intake and preference.*

Bolles, R. C. (1975). *Learning theory.* New York: Holt, Rinehart and Winston.

Costa, G., & Donaldson, S. S. (1979). Effects of cancer and cancer treatment on the nutrition of the host. *New England Journal of Medicine, 300,* 1471–1474.

Garcia, J., Ervin, F. R., & Koelling, R. A. (1966). Learning with prolonged delay of reinforcement. *Psychonomic Science, 5,* 121–122.

Garcia, J., Hankins, W. G., & Rusiniak, K. W. (1974). Behavioral regulation of the milieu interne in man and rat. *Science, 185,* 824–831.

Goodlad, G. A. J. (1964). Protein metabolism and tumor growth. In H. N. Munro and J. B. Allison (Eds.), *Mammalian protein metabolism* (Vol. II). New York: Academic Press.

Harper, A. E., Benevenga, N. J., & Wohlhueter, R. M. (1970). Effects of ingestion of disproportionate amounts of amino acids. *Physiological Review, 50,* 428–558.

Krause, R., James, J. H., Ziparo, V., & Fischer, J. E. (1979). Brain tryptophan and the neoplastic anorexia-cachexia syndrome. *Cancer, 44,* 1003–1008.

Lawson, D. H., Richmond, A., Nixon, D. W., & Rudman, D. (1982). Metabolic approaches to cancer cachexia. *Annual Review of Nutrition, 2,* 277–301.

Mordes, J. P., & Rossini, A. A. (1981). Tumor-induced anorexia in the Wistar rat. *Science, 213,* 565–567.

Morrison, S. D. (1975). Control of food intake during growth of a Walker 256 carcinosarcoma. *Cancer Research, 33,* 526–528.

Morrison, S. D. (1976). Control of food intake in cancer cachexia: a challenge and a tool. *Physiology and Behavior, 17,* 705–714.

Ohnuma, T., & Holland, J. F. (1977). Nutritional consequences of cancer chemotherapy and immunotherapy. *Cancer Research, 37,* 2395–2406.

Revusky, S. H., & Bedarf, E. W. (1967). Association of illness with prior ingestion of novel foods. *Science, 155,* 219–220.

Rogers, Q. R., & Leung, P. M. B. (1977). The control of food intake: When and how are amino acids involved? In M. R. Kare & O. Maller (Eds.), *The chemical senses and nutrition.* New York: Academic Press.

Rozin, P., & Kalat, J. W. (1971). Specific hungers and poison avoidance as adaptive specializations of learning. *Psychological Review, 78,* 459–486.

Schein, P. S., MacDonald, J. S., Waters, C., & Haidak, D. (1975). Nutritional complications of cancer and its treatment. *Seminars in Oncology, 2,* 337–347.

Treneer, C. M., & Bernstein, I. L. (1981). Learned aversions in rats fed a tryptophan-free diet. *Physiology and Behavior, 27,* 757–760.

Wu, C. & Bauer, J. M. (1960). A study of free amino acids and of glutamine synthesis in tumor-bearing rats. *Cancer Research, 20,* 848–857.

5 Radiation-Induced Taste Aversions in Rats and Humans

James C. Smith*
Judith T. Blumsack
Florida State University

F. S. Bilek, M. D.
Tallahassee Memorial Regional Medical Center

In 1955 Garcia, Kimeldorf and Koelling published a paper in *Science* which has had far reaching implications for many aspects of behavioral science. One of many important conclusions of that paper was that ionizing radiation could act as an unconditioned stimulus, radically altering the drinking behavior of laboratory rats. Animals which ingested a saccharin flavored water while being exposed to gamma rays from a cobalt 60 source avoided the saccharin flavor in subsequent saccharin-water preference tests. With the proper control groups, these investigators demonstrated that laboratory rats could learn to avoid a distinct taste which had been paired with the whole body irradiation. Many studies from Garcia's and others' laboratories manipulated parameters of this radiation-induced conditioning and furthered our understanding about the limitations and the physiological mechanisms underlying this association between tastes and irradiation. Although criticisms were abundant because this phenomenon was found to challenge the current thinking about learning, no scientific investigation refuted the original finding that tastes associated with irradiation were subsequently avoided. Concurrently with the irradiation work, a large literature began to grow which showed that a wide variety of drugs could also be used to condition taste aversions. Observations of drug-induced aversions had been made quite early (Garcia & Hankins, 1977), but it was not until after the Garcia, Kimeldorf and Koelling paper in 1955 that they were subjected to systematic observation with controls such as those used by Garcia et al.

Although there was an early interest in the application of drug-induced taste aversion learning to the treatment of alcoholism, it was not until the middle of the

*My sincere thanks go to Donald J. Kimeldorf, who taught me more than he will ever know.

1970s, some 20 years after the original Garcia et al. paper, that the National Cancer Institute began to request proposals to study the possible role of chemotherapy and irradiation-induced taste aversions in the dietary habits of patients with neoplastic diseases (see Chapter 1). As DeWys and Kisner (1982) have recently pointed out, some attention needs to be given to the antineoplastic therapies themselves as potential contributors to the decreased caloric intake so often seen in the cancer patient.

In our laboratory we have initiated a study of radiation-induced taste aversion as it may affect the human radiotherapy patient. We asked the question "are inadvertent radiation-induced taste aversions being conditioned because various tastants are experienced too close to radiation exposure?" The work has taken two approaches: (1) we have tried to develop a more adequate animal model for studying the role of conditioned taste aversion in the human patient, (2) we have attempted to directly condition a taste aversion in cancer radiotherapy patients and to develop procedures for accessing the impact of potential learned taste aversion on the dietary habits of these patients.

THE ANIMAL MODEL

The Basic Model

The basic demonstration for radiation-induced saccharin aversion which we use differs only slightly from the original Garcia, Kimeldorf and Koelling design. The saccharin flavored water is presented before the irradiation and the duration of the exposure is considerably shorter in our procedure. The procedure and data described in an earlier paper (Spector, Smith & Hollander, 1981) will serve as an example of the basic design which we have used. The rats were housed in individual cages and accustomed to receiving their water ration for ten minutes in the early morning. The conditioning group received saccharin flavored water (.1% sodium saccharin) for 10 minutes and were then transported to the Cobalt room where the animals received a whole body exposure to gamma rays for 33.4 minutes. The exposure was measured in air by a Victoreen Thimble Chamber to be 100r. For comparison, the LD 50 for Sprague-Dawley rats (i.e., the dose that is lethal for about 50% of the rats exposed to it) is about 750r (Casarett, 1968). The measure of aversion was like that of Garcia et al. (1955), i.e., a daily water vs. saccharin preference test which was continued over days until a recovery to normal saccharin drinking was observed. Many taste aversion experiments which followed the Garcia et al. (1955) paper measured aversion by some relatively short-term preference test. We thought it was important, in the animal model, to measure the aversion both by its magnitude and its duration. If these aversions were short lived, we would be less interested in their role in the eating behavior of radiotherapy patients. Garcia et al. (1955) found the aversion to last over fifty days which is a significant period in a rat's life.

We also followed the example of Garcia et al. (1955) and demonstrated that it is the pairing of the saccharin and the gamma rays which results in the long lasting aversion. Control groups which received saccharin and sham exposure, water and gamma exposure, and water and sham exposure on the "conditioning day" were included in the study. An illustration of these groups and typical first day preference scores from our data are presented in Fig. 5.1. The recovery from the aversion of the saccharin-radiation group can be seen in Fig. 5.2. The lack of any learned aversion in the three control groups can also be seen in this figure. Thus, this experiment supports the same conclusion as the original Garcia et al. (1955) study, i.e., the pairing of a normally preferred taste substance with a single sublethal exposure to ionizing radiation results in a profound and rather long lasting aversion to that tastant. Mere exposure to the gamma rays does not result in any aversion. In classical conditioning language, the conditioned stimulus (saccharin flavored water) when paired with the unconditioned stimulus (gamma rays) results in a conditioned aversion to the flavored water.

Human radiotherapy patients seldom receive whole body irradiation, they normally receive more than one exposure, and they do not necessarily (it has been our experience that they are not even likely to) consume novel tastants before they are exposed. For an appropriate animal model for the radiotherapy

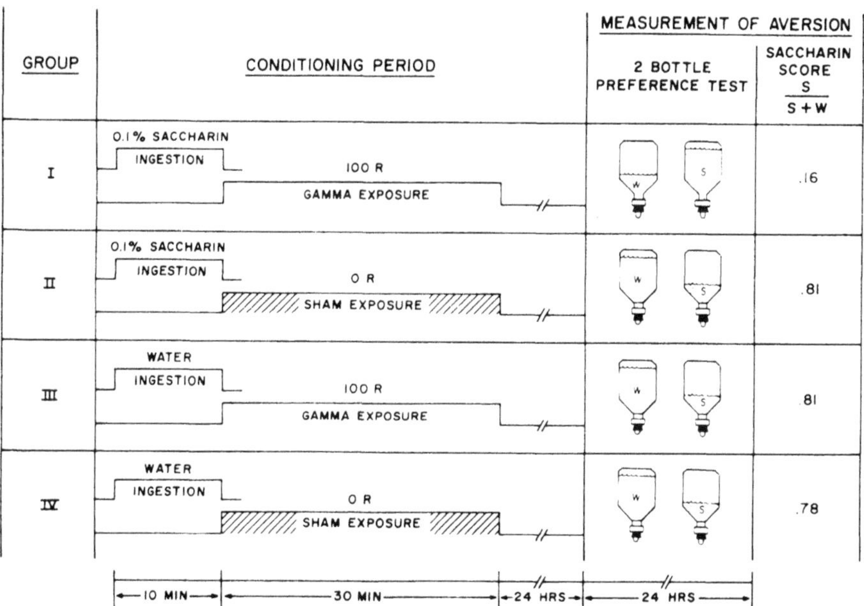

FIG. 5.1. A schematic diagram of our experimental design. The resulting saccharin scores (taken from Spector, Smith, & Hollander, 1981) are typical of almost all radiation-induced taste aversion experiments.

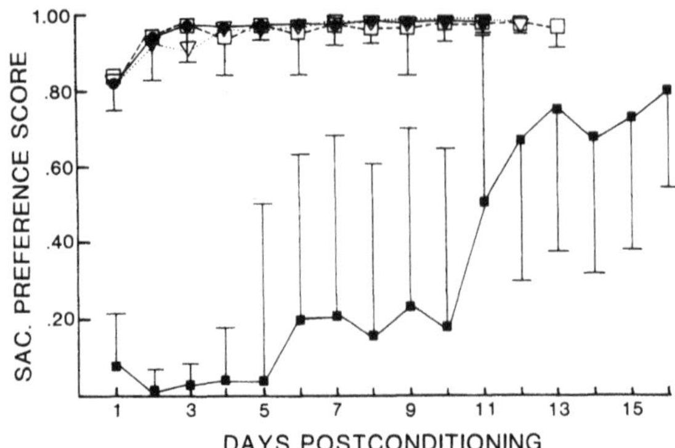

FIG. 5.2. Recovery from saccharin aversion is shown where median saccharin preference scores are plotted as a function of postconditioning test days. The group which received saccharin paired with radiation (solid squares) shows the average gradual recovery from the conditioned aversion. The control groups described in Fig. 5.1 show no aversion at any time to the saccharin.

patient we needed to demonstrate a conditioned taste aversion in a rat which was thoroughly familiar with the tastant and which was given several partial body exposures. If these manipulations were to result in a profound and long lasting aversion it would give more impetus to test for learned aversions in the radiotherapy patient.

Partial Body Exposures

From the literature it is apparent that many of these manipulations have been made, but not all in the same animal. Garcia and Kimeldorf (1960) have demonstrated that aversions can be conditioned with partial body exposures. In fact, they showed that abdominal exposure was more sensitive in conditioning the aversion than was head, thoracic or pelvic exposure. Smith, Hollander and Spector (1981) tested the effects of head, abdomen, or whole body exposure with the procedure described above, i.e., 20 minutes of saccharin followed by gamma ray exposure, and used a 10-minute saccharin drinking aversion test on the next day. Their results, which replicated Garcia and Kimeldorf's (1960) findings, are shown in Fig. 5.3. The extinction curves for the 200r exposure of head and abdomen can be seen in Fig. 5.4. These data show that the recovery from head exposure is much more rapid than that from abdominal exposure. In fact, tests on other rats receiving 200r abdominal exposure revealed that they had not recovered normal saccharin drinking after more than 50 days of post-exposure testing.

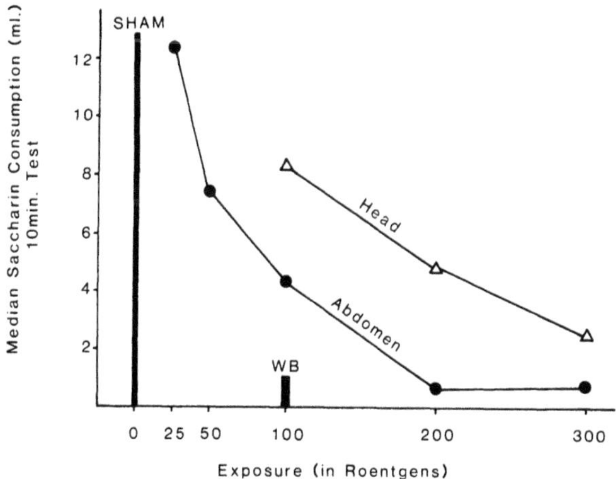

FIG. 5.3. Median saccharin consumption on the postconditioning 10-minute single-bottle test for groups receiving whole body (WB), head or abdominal exposure at the exposures described.

Effects of Prior Saccharin Experiences

Numerous investigators have shown that familiarity with the taste solution prior to conditioning day markedly attentuates the magnitude and duration of the learned aversion (e.g., Smith, 1971). This was certainly true with our procedure. Rats given ten preconditioning sessions (10 minutes each) with the saccharin flavored water showed little, if any, conditioning unless they were given 200 r whole body exposure. This is illustrated in Fig. 5.5. Recovery from the aversion was also much more rapid in the rats which were familiar with the saccharin. It can be seen in Fig. 5.6 that the recovery in the 300r exposed group is quite

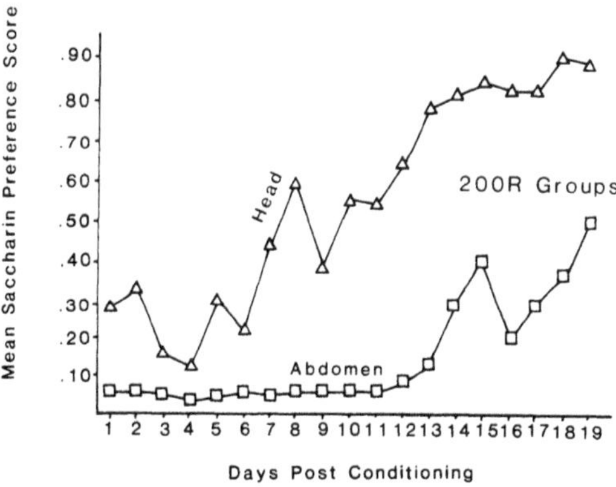

FIG. 5.4. Recovery from a radiation-induced taste aversion is seen where median saccharin preference scores are plotted as a function of postirradiation test days for groups which received 200r exposures to either the head or abdominal area.

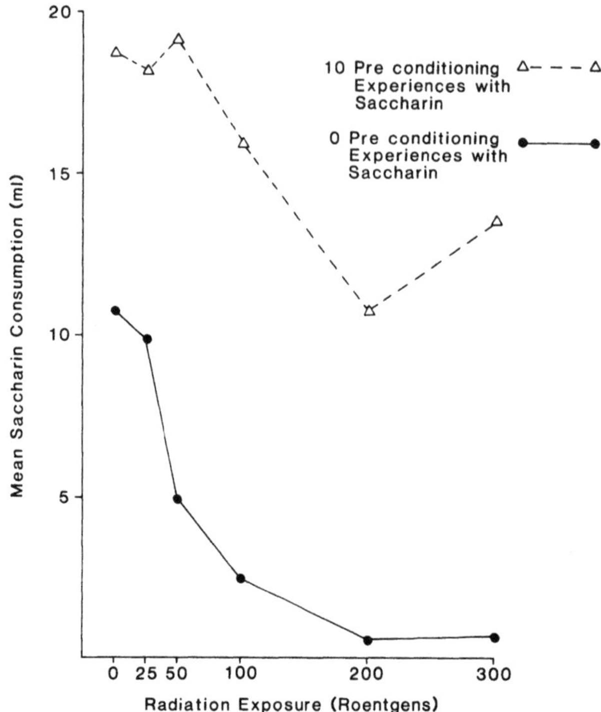

FIG. 5.5. Mean saccharin consumption in a ten-minute postconditioning test as a function of radiation exposure.

profound as compared to the rats with no prior saccharin experience. In this 300r group the initial conditioning of the saccharin experienced animals was as strong as that for the taste naive rats. The attenuating effects of preconditioning saccharin habituation are so strong that the animal model would predict that learned taste aversions in radiotherapy patients would be trivial unless they ate novel foods. One must remember, however, that the results were from experiments where only one conditioning trial was administered.

Multiple Radiation Exposures

Garcia and Koelling (1967) reported over fifteen years ago that three conditioning trials with saccharin and x–rays could overcome a lifetime of experience with saccharin. In order to test the effects of multiple saccharin-whole body radiation pairings in rats familiar with the tastant on the long-term recovery from a saccharin aversion, we compared groups of rats that had: (1) ten habituations to saccharin and one saccharin-radiation pairing; (2) no habituation to saccharin and one saccharin-radiation pairing; and (3) ten habituations to saccharin followed by

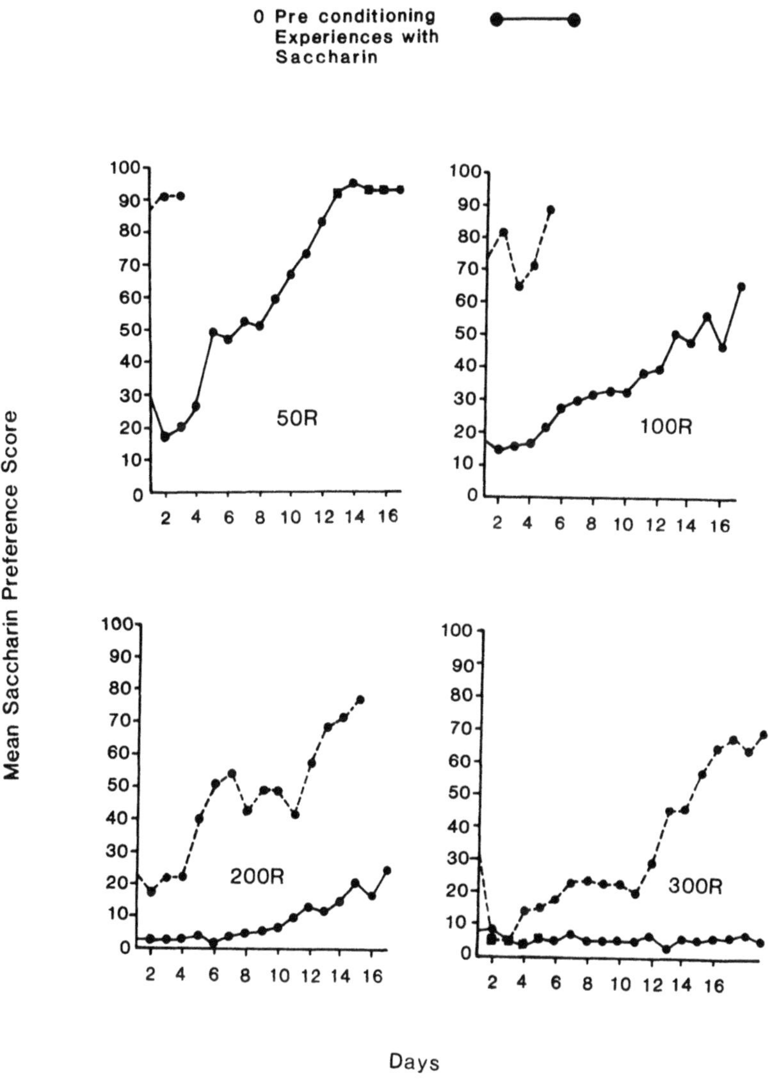

FIG. 5.6. Mean saccharin preference score plotted as a function of postconditioning testing days for groups receiving 50r, 100r, 200r or 300r exposures.

three saccharin-radiation pairings. The long term recovery from the aversions conditioned in these groups is illustrated in Fig. 5.7. Here it can be seen that 10 habituations to saccharin followed by one saccharin-radiation pairing resulted in no conditioning. Rats treated identically, but given three saccharin-radiation

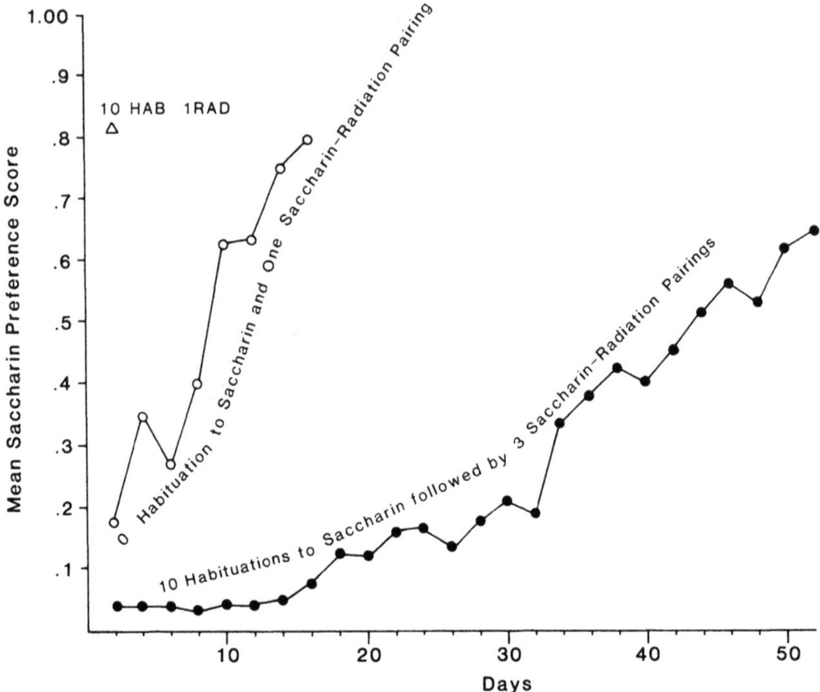

FIG. 5.7. Mean saccharin preference score as a function of postconditioning testing days. Recovery from aversion is compared among groups which received 10 habituations to saccharin followed by three conditioning trials (solid circles), zero habituation trials and one conditioning trial (open circles), and 10 habituations to saccharin followed by one conditioning trial (open triangles).

pairings on three consecutive days, showed a profound aversion which was not overcome in more than fifty days.

The next step was to test rats with multiple partial body exposures during the conditioning trials. All of these rats had received 10 daily habituation trials to the saccharin flavored water. Rats were exposed to 100r to the head or the abdomen. Each conditioning day they were given 10 minutes of saccharin followed by the 100r gamma exposure until their 10 minute saccharin intake mean was not significantly different from a criterion group mean. The "criterion" group had no experience with saccharin prior to the conditioning day, when they received a single 100r whole body exposure following 10 minutes of saccharin ingestion. The "criterion" was the amount of saccharin they consumed in a single bottle test on the day following conditioning. As can be seen in Fig. 5.8, this criterion value was about 4 ml. The abdomen group took only three trials before they were "conditioned" by the criterion described above. The head group took five pair-

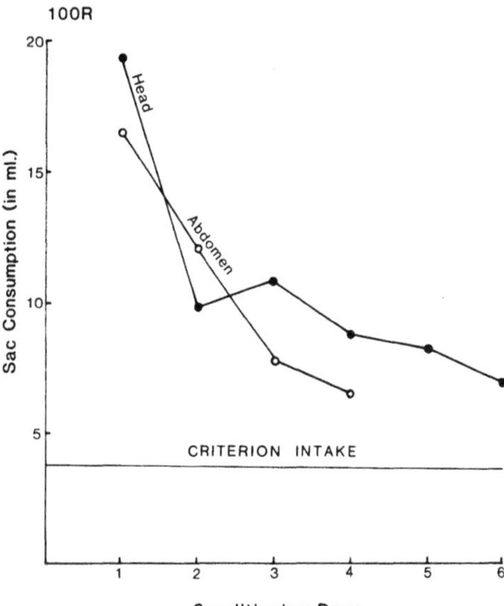

FIG. 5.8. Mean saccharin consumption in a ten-minute drinking period as a function of number of conditioning days. Animals exposed to the abdomen were not statistically different from the criterion intake level (see text) after three conditioning trials (open circles) and those exposed to the head took five trials (closed circles) to reach the criterion.

ings of the saccharin and irradiation to reach the same criterion. The last data point for each group was not followed by irradiation. Control animals received either water and irradiation or saccharin and sham irradiation on conditioning day. The partial recovery from these conditioning trials is seen in Fig. 5.9. The combined control animals showed no sign of aversion. The recovery to normal saccharin drinking for both groups was incomplete even after 50 days. The course of recovery for these groups was not statistically different. One could conclude that multiple partial body exposures during conditioning trials with rats that were not naive to saccharin resulted in profound and long lasting aversions to the tastants. It also appears that head irradiation can be as effective as abdominal irradiation if enough saccharin–radiation pairings have been made. This latter conclusion is limited, however, to this particular 100r exposure. The final step in developing our current animal model was to compare head, abdominal and whole body exposures with several radiation levels in rats that were thoroughly familiar with saccharin.

Eighty-one male rats were given ten days of habituation trials (10 minutes/per day) to saccharin flavored water. After drinking saccharin for 10 minutes on the conditioning day they were confined to plexiglas tubes and given either a whole body, head, or abdominal exposure to gamma rays. Each of the three groups was further subdivided into three groups which received either a 25r, 50r or 200r exposure (N = 9 in each group). Conditioning trials were continued for each group until the mean fluid consumption during the CS period was less than 20% of that consumed on the first conditioning day. In order to avoid severe depriva-

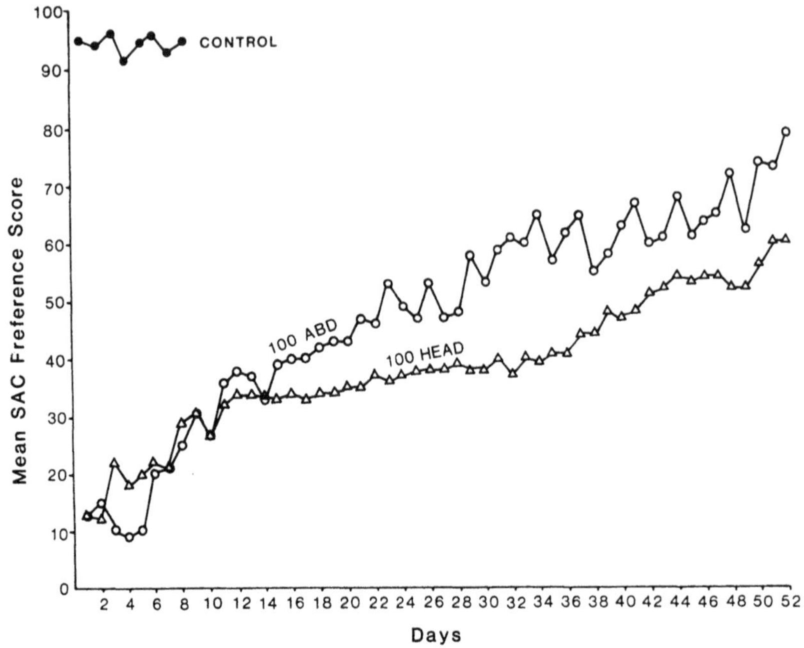

FIG. 5.9. Mean saccharin preference score as a function of postconditioning testing days. Recovery for rats conditioned with radiation to the head (open triangles) and to the abdomen (open circles) followed the same course and was not complete after 52 days. Data for control rats that received either saccharin-sham trials or water-radiation trials were combined (closed circles).

tion during these multiple conditioning trials, all rats were given a 10 minute water supplement about five hours after conditioning each day. Four of the groups failed to reach the conditioning criterion and conditioning trials were discontinued on these groups after two weeks of exposures. Table 5.1 shows the number of days for conditioning in each of the groups.

From Table 5.1, one would conclude that 25r to whole body, abdomen, or head and 50r to the head was not a strong enough dose to condition the rats. As expected whole body exposure took fewer trials than did abdominal exposure, and abdominal exposure was more sensitive than head exposure.

Once the conditioning criterion was met (or after 14 days of CS–US pairings if conditioning did not occur by this time), 24-hour two-bottle preference testing was initiated. The mean saccharin preference scores for the first 24-hour postexposure preference test are presented in Fig. 5.10. From these data it can be seen that conditioning did occur at the 25r level for the whole body and abdominal groups in spite of the failure to meet the conditioning criterion. At the 50r level all three groups were conditioned, but in the abdominal and whole body groups

TABLE 5.1
The Number of Pairings of Saccharin With Cobalt 60 Exposure for Each Treatment Condition

	Number of Conditioning Days		
	Whole Body	Abdomen	Head
25 r	14	14	14
50 r	3	5	14
200 r	2	3	4

the conditioning was stronger. At the 200r level all groups became well conditioned. The recovery from these aversions is plotted in Fig. 5.11. Here it can be seen that whole body exposure generally resulted in stronger conditioning than abdominal exposure and head exposure except at the 200r level. The recovery to normal drinking for the whole body exposure groups does not seem to depend on the daily exposure. This is also probably true for the abdominal groups. For the head groups, there was considerable difference in the time for recovery. Initially, the 25r group showed almost no aversion. The 50r group showed some aversion

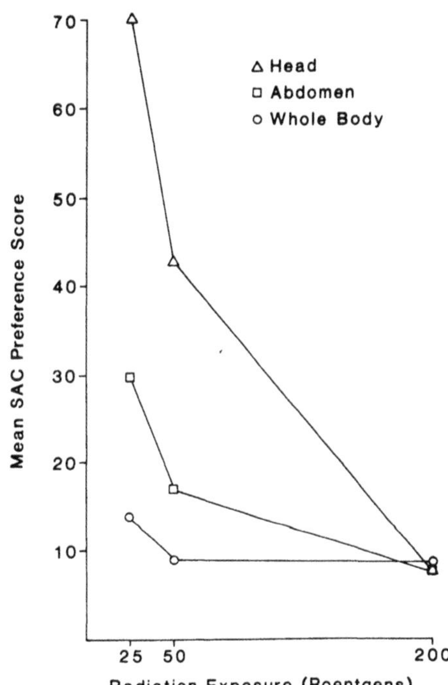

FIG. 5.10. Mean saccharin preference score as a function of radiation exposure for rats treated with head (open triangles), abdomen (open squares) or whole body (open circles) gamma ray exposures.

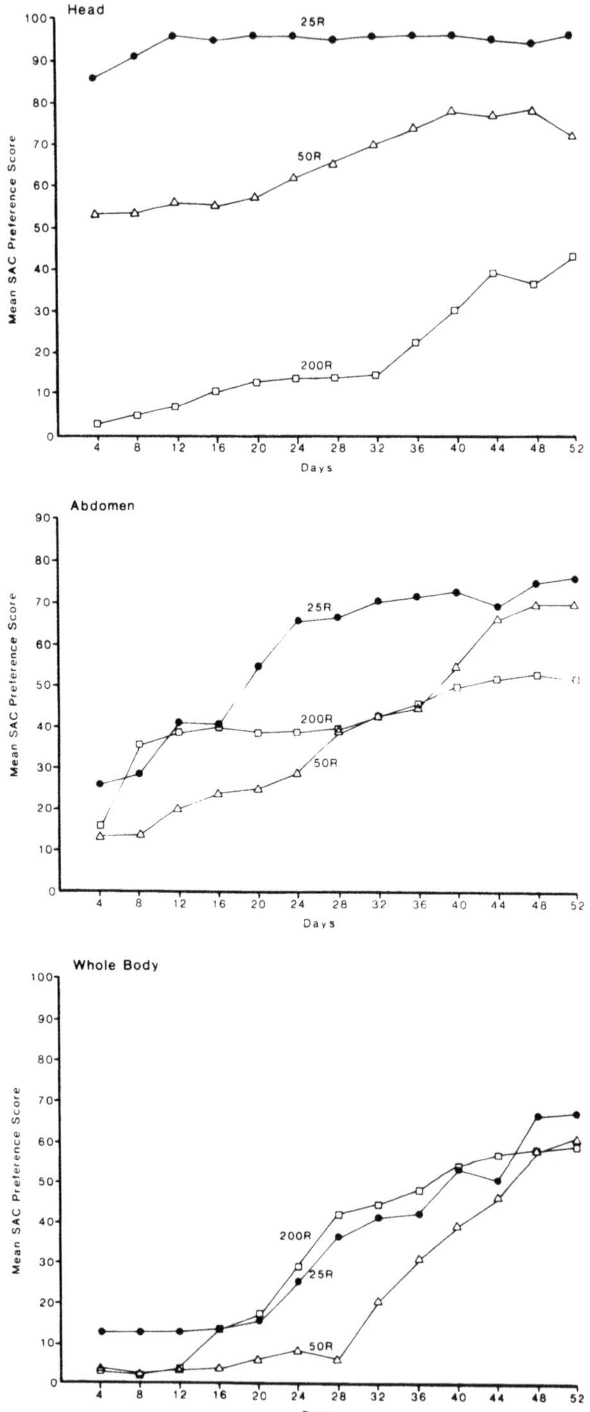
Head
25R
50R
200R
Mean SAC Preference Score
Days
Abdomen
25R
200R
50R
Mean SAC Preference Score
Days
Whole Body
200R
25R
50R
Mean SAC Preference Score
Days

and a slower recovery rate. The 200r group showed about the same recovery rate as the 50r group, but the initial aversion was much more profound. Even after 52 days the 50r group is not completely recovered and the 200r group has barely reached a point of indifference. In the head groups, the difference between the 50 and 200r groups cannot be accounted for by the total radiation exposure. The 200r group received a total of 800r in four days when the 50r group received 700r in 14 days. There seems to be something qualitatively different about the 200r group and head irradiation, a point we will return to later in the chapter.

It can be concluded from the animal model studies that rats irradiated under conditions similar to those experienced by radiotherapy patients indeed do develop profound and long lasting aversions to a familiar tastant. The next step in our program was to demonstrate taste aversion in a radiotherapy patient.

TASTE AVERSION CONDITIONING IN HUMANS

Thirty-four adults ranging in age from 18 to 78 years volunteered as subjects for an experiment to test for radiation-induced taste aversion in humans. Twenty of the subjects were radiotherapy patients at the Tallahassee Memorial Regional Medical Center. These outpatients were receiving abdominal or pelvic radiation for a variety of different neoplastic diseases. None of them had had prior radiation or chemotherapy treatments. The other 14 subjects were normal adults with no known neoplastic diseases (Smith, Blumsack, Bilek, Spector, Hollander & Baker, 1984). They were selected from a group of nonfaculty employees at the Florida State University and had no knowledge about the project at the hospital. Ten of the radiotherapy patients were informed that they were part of a study to investigate taste preferences and eating patterns during the period when they were receiving radiation treatments. They were informed that they would be asked to answer questions about their diet, to respond to a rating scale about certain foods and to select a fruit juice for refreshment during their interview. These patients were offered a choice of apple, orange or grape juice 15 to 60 minutes prior to their first irradiation. The patient selected one juice and indicated the amount he or she wished to consume. This averaged 201 ml and ranged from 89 to 400 ml. On each subsequent treatment day during the interview the patient was offered only the same juice that was selected on the first treatment day. This group served as a tastant-radiation group. The rating scale was a modification of a scale developed by Peryam and Pilgrim (1957). A nine point rating from "dislike extremely" to "like extremely" was used for each of the eleven following substances: apple juice, fried chicken, coffee, mashed potatoes, orange juice, cooked carrots, sweet rolls, grape juice, lima beans, white rice, and

FIG. 5.11. Mean saccharin preference scores as a function of postconditioning testing days for the radiation exposures and treatment sites indicated.

ham. The rating scale was presented to the patient for completion during approximately 40% of the interviews. From this procedure we could measure on each treatment day the quantity of juice consumed prior to irradiation and we could periodically measure the patient's attitude toward that particular juice and toward 10 other tastants.

The fourteen normal adults were treated in a similar fashion as the patients except that they received no irradiation. They were told that they were part of a study in which we were studying eating behavior in cancer patients and that they were to serve as a nondisease control group. They were also told that we would ask them to complete a rating scale about food and that they would receive a refreshment of their choice during the interview period. These subjects were seen daily for 15 consecutive working days. This group served as a tastant-no irradiation control.

The second group of ten radiotherapy patients was offered no juice or rating scale. The patients were selected from a larger group which we had been interviewing daily throughout radiotherapy. They were selected because they were being treated in the abdominal or pelvic region and because they indicated in their interviews that they were regular drinkers of some particular, distinctive tasting liquid, such as orance juice or others. This tastant, however, was not systematically consumed by the patient at any particular time and definitely not during the interview period prior to irradiation. On each treatment day these patients were interviewed either before or after their radiation treatment, so that their dietary intake since the last interview could be recorded. They served as an irradiated group which received no tastant close in time to therapy.

All patients in the tastant-irradiation group developed an aversion to their particular juice. Whether it was apple, grape or orange juice the amount requested and the amount consumed dropped radically after the first treatment day. In fact, all but one of the patients refused to taste the juice at all after from one to 13 pairings. The average number of pairings until this complete cessation was six. It appeared that the demand characteristics of the procedure and not a desire for grape juice kept the 10th patient drinking a small quantity throughout radiotherapy. He was convinced that the doctor wanted him to drink the grape juice for therapeautic reasons. The data for one patient who showed an aversion to grape juice and a change in attitude toward grape juice are seen in Fig. 5.12. The amount of grape juice consumed dropped rapidly to zero and he continued to refuse any of this tastant throughout the therapy period. It can be seen that his rating scale indicated a similar growing dislike for grape juice. His ratings of the other foods and juices were constant. Consistency in rating the nonconditioned tastants was also seen in the other nine patients. Although they all showed the marked change in behavior toward their selected juice, they did not all show a change on their rating scale, as did the patient illustrated in Fig. 5.12. In fact only four of the 10 patients indicated a decreased preference for their particular juice on this rating scale. Several of the patients rated their juice as "like extremely"

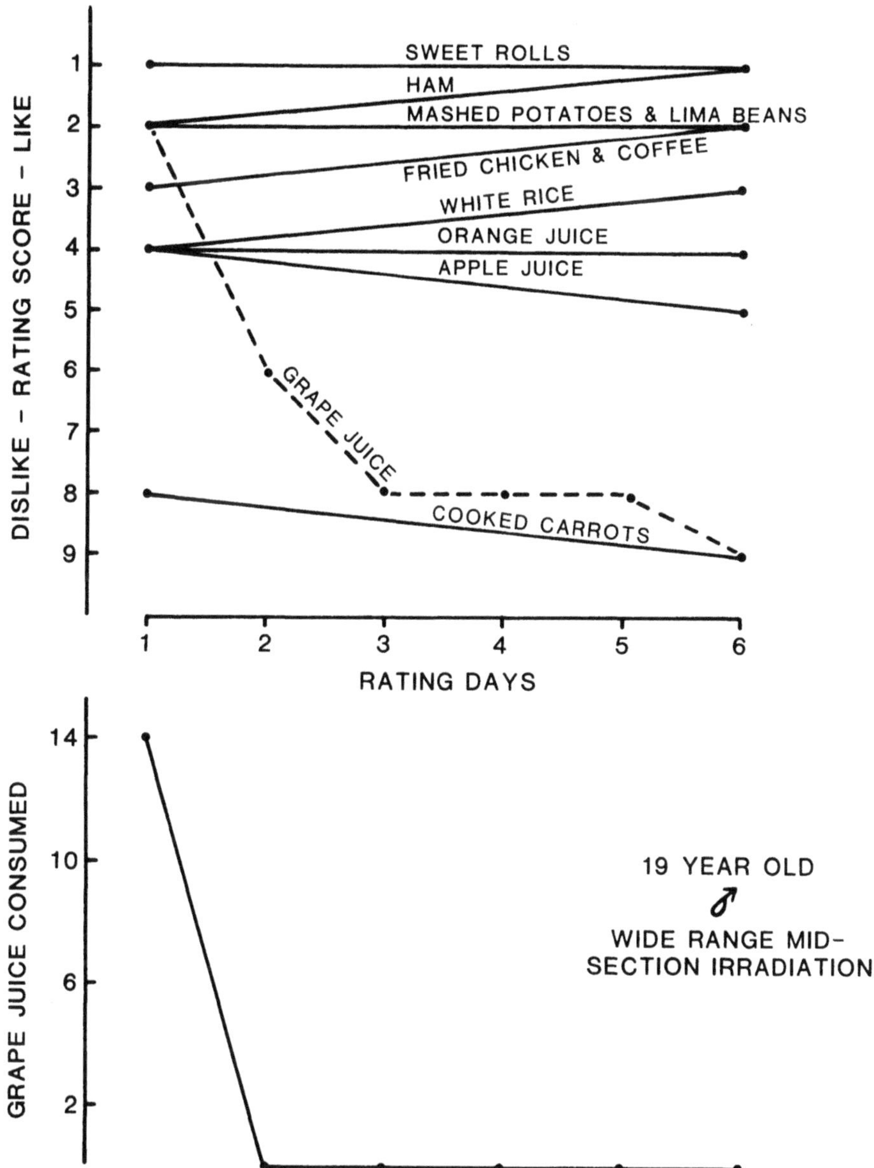

FIG. 5.12. Upper panel: Rating scores from like extremely (1) to dislike extremely (9) as a function of six rating days distributed throughout the course of radiotherapy. For all of the tastants except grape juice, only the first and last rating days are recorded. Lower panel: Grape juice consumption as a function of the same rating days indicated in the upper panel.

and at the same time would not drink it. These data, although preliminary, are interesting in themselves in showing the lack of correlation between the verbal report and the eating behavior of the patient.

The normal tastant-no irradiation subjects showed no signs of decreasing their juice intake. Eleven of the subjects were extremely consistent in the amount they drank each day and the other three subjects showed a slight increase over the fifteen day period. There were no significant changes in their rating scales for any of the tastants during the fifteen day period. Only one subject changed as much as two units on the nine point scale of any tastant. These data show that continued daily drinking of these fruit juices does not result in a decrease in amount consumed.

The analysis of the data from the irradiation control group was somewhat different. From the interviews with these ten patients we found that three of these patients were regular orange juice drinkers, one drank Gatorade, one drank grapefruit juice, one drank orange soda, one drank Koolade and three drank milk. These beverages were imbibed regularly throughout the course of radiation therapy at various times of the day. They were not consumed close in time to treatment. The data from this group suggest that pelvic or abdominal radiation itself does not necessarily result in a decrease in the intake of flavored liquids.

The two "control groups" are not comparable to the experimental group in all aspects, and our data cannot be considered definitive. However, when taken together there is considerable evidence that supports a learned aversion interpretation of the data obtained from the patients where the distinctive tastant was paired with irradiation. These results concern only a short term aversion and no tests were run to examine how long this aversion would last or to study what effect this aversion could have on the overall eating patterns of the patients.

Including the 10 patients we saw in the no tastant-irradiation group above, we interviewed approximately 60 radiotherapy patients about their daily dietary intakes. They ranged in age from 18 to 78 and represented a broad spectrum of disease types and stages. They also differed widely in their prior medical histories. We interviewed them on each treatment day and with many patients we were able to gain additional information in follow-up interviews. We paid special attention to indications of learned food aversions, i.e., did any of the patients show specific aversions to foods which they ate close in time to exposure.

Indications of learned taste aversion were observed in a few of these patients from their comments about food preference and appetite changes. Four of the patients, all of whom were treated in the abdominal area, reported a strong and specific aversion to a particular food consumed close in time to a radiation treatment. These aversions lasted from several weeks to several months. Although we observed many other changes in food preference behavior, perceived taste sensitivity, and appetite, these changes did not appear to be radiation-induced learned food aversions.

In the animal work, we systematically have paired tastants with radiation exposure to determine the conditions under which learned taste aversions occur. It appears from the present work that aversions can be conditioned in humans undergoing irradiation if a tastant is systematically paired with the exposures to radiation. It is quite likely that the varied eating and drinking patterns of human radiotherapy patients provide considerable protection against the formation of learned taste aversion in the routine course of radiotherapy. One would assume that there would be little taste aversion conditioned in a rat if the animal received numerous trials of tastant with no irradiation and/or trials with no tastant and irradiation interspersed with tastant-irradiation trials.

In conclusion, our data suggest that aversive conditioning is a possible contributing factor to eating problems in cancer radiation patients, but that this contribution does not seem to be overwhelming in magnitude. However, since we know that aversive conditioning can lead to dietary problems, it might be useful for oncologists and radiotherapists to be aware of these data in treating their patients. In some cases it may be advisable to discourage patients from eating (particularly new foods or beverages) close in time to radiotherapy treatments. The obvious question is: "What is 'close in time'"?. One can only speculate about this question in the work with radiotherapy patients, but there are considerable data on this question from the rat studies which will be considered in the next section.

HOW TO PREVENT RADIATION-INDUCED TASTE AVERSIONS

There are several ways that radiation-induced taste aversion could be avoided. The first, and most obvious, is to insure that no tastant is "paired" with irradiation. It was stated in the earlier discussion of the animal research that radiation without the tastant produced no saccharin aversion. This statement must be qualified because one of the early findings in this research was that radiation (the US) could be given either before or after the tastant (the CS) and yet this "loose pairing" would still result in the conditioned aversion to saccharin. Although research on this topic has been quite difficult for the traditional learning theorist to accept, it has been shown that in the rat the CS could precede the US by as long as six hours and still produce significant aversion (Smith & Roll, 1967). In addition, it has been shown that the US could precede the CS by 6 hours and conditioning would result (Smith, 1971). In fact, this postexposure condition (i.e., where the US precedes the CS) proved in many cases to result in even stronger initial conditioning than the more traditional CS–US pairing (Barker & Smith, 1974). Many studies showed that if the rat drank saccharin either several hours before or after irradiation, it would develop an aversion to saccharin.

These studies all were done with a 100r whole-body exposure. No systematic studies which combined partial body exposures, multiple exposures, or the novelty of the tastant with the manipulation of the temporal relations of the saccharin and radiation have been done. Furthermore, in the studies which manipulated the CS–US relationship no measures were taken to see how long the aversion lasted. Preliminary studies from this laboratory indicate that if the whole-body irradiation exposure was increased from 100r to 300r, that the irradiation could precede the saccharin by 24 hours or more and still produce saccharin aversion. Considerably more data must be collected before any speculation could be made regarding a time safety factor for radiotherapy patients.

A second approach to prevent radiation-induced taste aversions in cancer radiotherapy patients would be to block the aversive aspect of the radiation exposure. There is some evidence from the animal literature about what the aversive aspects of the radiation exposure are and how to prevent the aversions. Hunt, Carroll, and Kimeldorf (1968) generated strong evidence that the aversive aspect of irradiation which resulted in taste aversion learning was humorally mediated. Their studies with parabiont pairs of rats (i.e., rats whose blood circulatory systems were surgically connected) showed that if one member of the pair drank saccharin while the partner was being irradiated, the saccharin-drinking rat would subsequently avoid the saccharin. Further, Garcia, Ervin and Koelling (1967) showed that rats that drank saccharin and were injected with serum from irradiated donors developed an aversion to the saccharin. Levy, Ervin, and Garcia (1970) were able to block the contractile response to irradiation in an *in vitro* gut preparation with an injection of chlortrimeton. In our laboratory we conducted behavioral tests to see if the humorally-mediated aversive substance which caused radiation-induced taste aversions was histamine (Levy, Carroll, Smith & Hofer, 1974). We were able to produce an aversion in rats which had tasted saccharin followed by an injection of histamine diphosphate. Rats which had been pretreated with chlorpheniramine, an active H_1 histamine antogonist, failed to develop a radiation-induced taste aversion. Tigan, an effective antimetic drug, did not block the formation of the radiation-induced taste aversion. Captializing on the fact that radiation-induced taste aversion can best be conditioned if the radiation precedes the saccharin drinking by 30–90 minutes, we injected the chlorphenirmine, exposed the rats to cobalt 60 and then gave the animals access to the saccharin until they consumed 10 ml of saccharin-flavored water. This avoided conditioning an aversion to chlorpheniramine; it is not possible to do "backward" conditioning with drug injections. Sessions (1975) and Cairnie and Leach (1982) have criticized this procedure and have failed to block radiation-induced taste aversion with chlorpheniramine when they followed the sequence of saccharin ingestion, chlorpheniramine injection, and irradiation. In both of their studies they produced saccharin aversions to the chlorpheniramine alone, so their failure to block the aversion may merely reflect an aversion to the chlorpheniramine. As Sessions has pointed out (1975), before the hypothesis that histamine release is responsible for radiation-induced taste aversion conditioning is tenable, the procedures for administration of the antihistamine must be clarified. Levy (1975) has shown stronger saccharin aversion in adrenalectomized rats than in control animals following a weak radiation exposure of 50r whole body. She speculated that adrenalectomized rats were more sensitive to histamine than normal rats. Furthermore, she showed that chlorpheniramine maleate could inhibit formalin-induced taste aversions and again postulated a histamine release as the basis of formalin-induced taste aversions. Needless to say, considerable research is needed with animals before the use of antihistamine is considered for human radiotherapy patients.

We have spent some time in studying the recovery of rats from radiation-induced taste aversion in order to develop ways to hasten the recovery process. In Fig. 5.2 of this chapter an extinction curve for aversion is illustrated based on the median scores for 32 rats. What is not seen here is the tremendous variability among the rats in rates of recovery. As Fig. 5.13 illustrates, a few of the animals recover from the aversion in two or three days (panel A), a few more in five to six days, and a few more in 11 days (panel B). For some the recovery is slower (panel C) and for some there is no recovery (panel D). In fact, the orderly median curve of Fig. 5.2 really reflects "how many rats have recovered by a certain time." Furthermore, when recovery starts, its course is rapid. This led us to speculate that some rats for some reason taste the saccharin and, receiving no bad effects, begin to taste it more and more. We tested this idea of recovery by allowing different groups of rats "saccharin alone" experience for varying times after conditioning to see if this hastened extinction of the aversion (Spector, Smith & Hollander, 1983). Figure 5.14 shows saccharin preference scores for a 24-hour test after conditioning and following a "saccharin alone" experience for 0, 3, 6, 12, 24, and 46 hours. It can be seen from the clear bars in the graph that the longer the saccharin-alone period following conditioning, the less the subsequent aversion. If the rat receives the saccharin alone for 24 hours after conditioning, there is no evidence for subsequent learned taste aversion. The finding is consistent with the idea of Revusky and Garcia (1980) that the one-bottle test creates a conflict situation for the fluid-deprived animal pitting the aversiveness of the saccharin against thirst. It is clear from these data that the profound and long-lasting taste aversion described earlier in this paper is at least in part the result of restricting the rat to a two-bottle preference test. When the rat has the option of drinking saccharin or not drinking at all, it chooses the former alternative and subsequently overcomes the aversion. It may be that human cancer radiotherapy patients, although not forced to ingest a substance they have developed an aversion to, may do so out of force of habit, e.g., the person may without thought sip coffee or eat toast at breakfast the day after radiotherapy even though on the previous day these substances were associated with the adverse consequences of radiotherapy. Discovering that the substance in question (e.g., the coffee or toast) was not followed by any adverse consequences, the person,

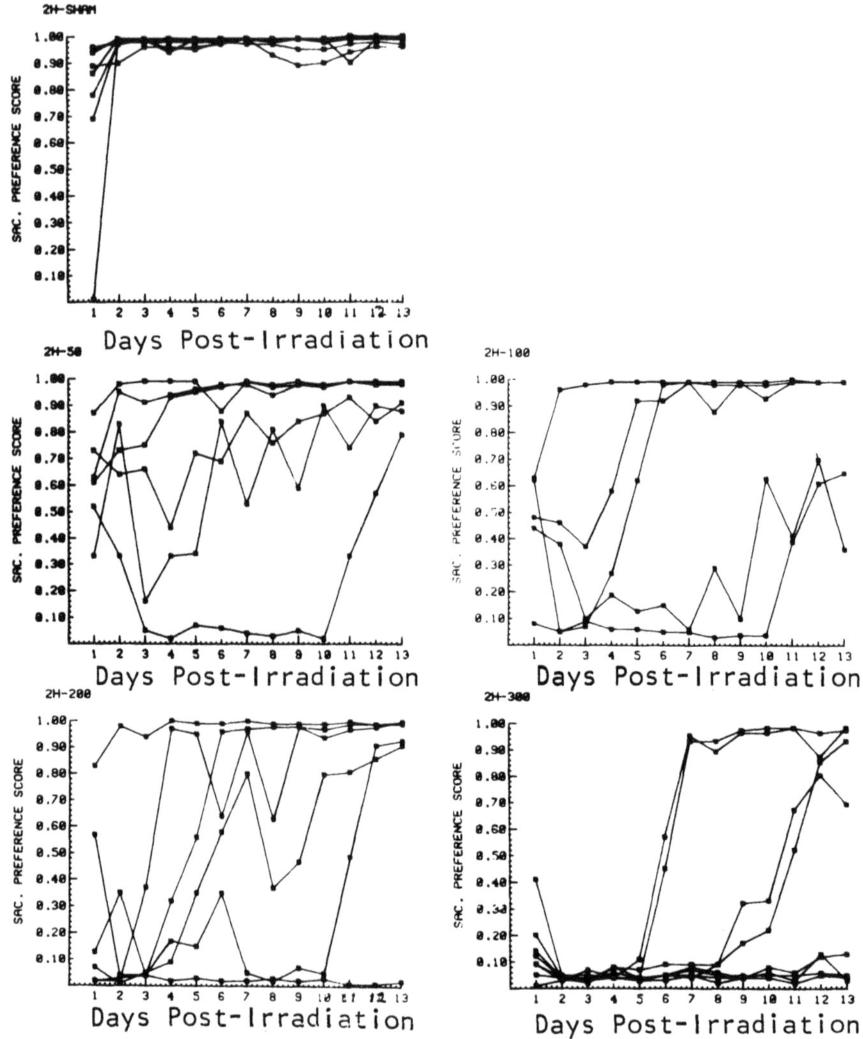

FIG. 5.13. In order to show the wide variability in recovering from a radiation-induced taste aversion conditioning, individual saccharin preference scores are plotted as a function of postconditioning test days for 32 rats, which all received identical conditioning treatment, i.e., 10 minutes of saccharin ingestion followed by a 100r whole-body exposure. The nine animals shown in panel A were recovered to normal saccharin drinking by Day 5. The six in panel B were recovered by Day 11 and the 18 rats in panel C showed a much more gradual recovery over the 16 testing days. The five rats in panel D showed no signs of recovery in 16 days.

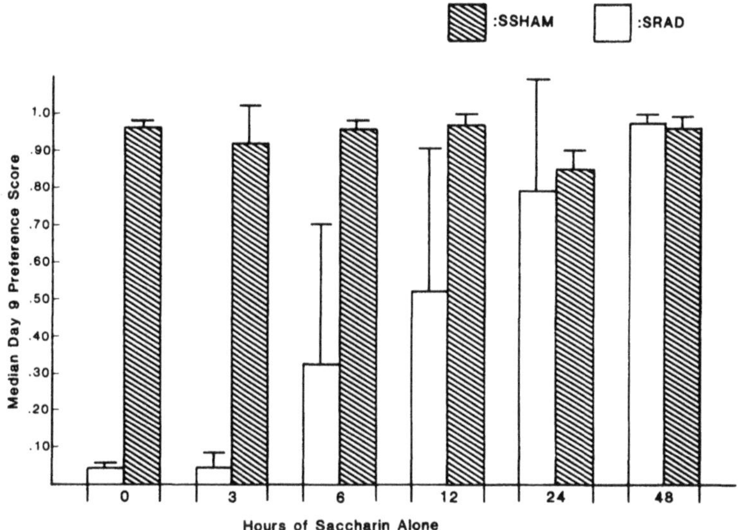

FIG. 5.14. Median saccharin preference scores for the first postirradiation preference test as a function of the amount of saccharin alone experience the different groups had after conditioning. The open bars are for groups of rats that had saccharin and radiation (SRAD) on conditioning day and the hatched bars are for groups of rats that received saccharin and sham exposure (S SHAM) on conditioning day.

like our rats, may quickly overcome any aversion that had been developed to the substance. Such a process would help to explain the fact that there appear to be relatively few taste aversions in cancer radiotherapy patients. However, it might be helpful to the radiotherapist to be aware of the possibility of the formation of learned taste aversions in his/her patients, especially in patients treated in the abdominal area, and to consider ways to minimize the aversive conditioning process.

FURTHER CONSIDERATIONS ABOUT RADIATION-INDUCED TASTE AVERSIONS

Whether one considers the role of radiation-induced taste aversions in cancer radiotherapy or merely addresses the problem as a basic research issue, there are many unresolved questions about the physiological basis of this unconditioned stimulus. Although the histamine hypothesis may be tenable for some levels of irradiation, it is most likely that many other factors are involved at the higher radiation doses. When a rat is given saccharin before a 300r exposure, the resulting aversion to the sweetened solution is much more profound and long lasting than the aversion from the conditioning with 100r exposure. Data for a single rat are presented in Fig. 5.15, where it can be seen that even after 23 days

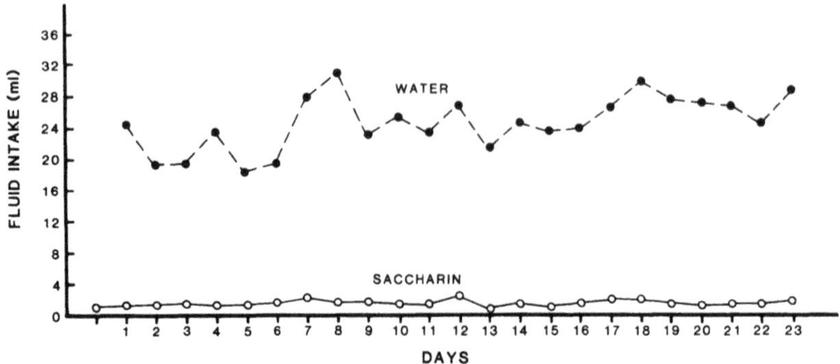

FIG. 5.15. Saccharin and water intake on 23 daily preference tests for one rat following a saccharin-300r radiation pairing. Water drinking averaged about 25 ml/day and saccharin drinking never exceeded 3 ml/day, indicating no signs of recovery from aversion.

there are no signs of a return to normal saccharin drinking. In fact, none of the many rats we tested ever drank more than three ml of saccharin during a 24-hour preference test after the 300r exposure. Similar results were obtained with abdominal exposure but not with head exposure as can be seen in Fig. 5.16. It is quite likely that the physiological basis for the aversion from a 300r exposure is qualitatively as well as quantitatively different from the 100r exposure. No attempts have been made yet to block these profound aversions with antihistamines.

Another issue involves several pecularities about taste aversions with head-only exposures. Although exposure of the head is *not* a *necessary* condition for forming a saccharin aversion with radiation exposure, there is evidence that head exposure can be an important and perhaps a facilitating factor in conditioning the aversion, as shown by the following studies.

Dinc and Smith (1966) reported that bilateral ablation of the olfactory bulbs resulted in a reduction of the magnitude of radiation-induced saccharin aversion.

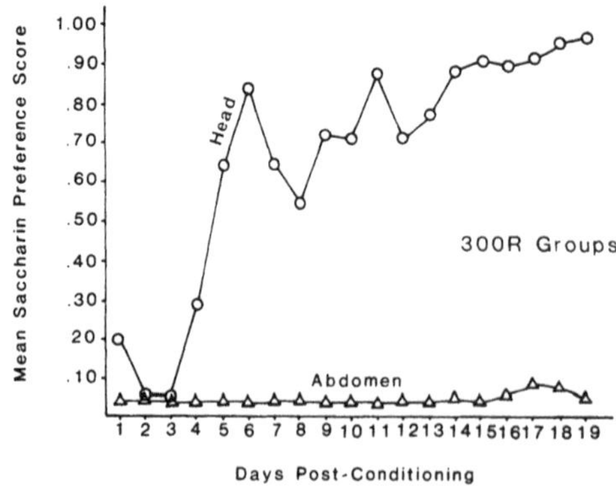

FIG. 5.16. Recovery from aversion (or lack thereof as seen in the abdominal exposed group) when median saccharin preference score is plotted as a function of 19 postconditioning preference test days.

One implication could be that olfaction plays some role in radiation-induced aversions. It is obvious, however, that removal of the olfactory bulbs could have effects other than anosmia. However, Reige (1968) reported that occlusion of the nasal passages inhibited the formation of the aversion. It is known that rats can detect the presence of ionizing radiation through the olfactory system if the exposure rate is high enough (Dinc & Smith, 1966; Cooper, Kimeldorf & McCarky, 1966), so it is possible that in the whole-body radiation-induced taste aversion experiments, stimulation of the olfactory system abets other physiological reactions resulting in a facilitated aversive response.

Smith, Hollander and Spector (1981) observed a marked difference in the recovery from radiation-induced taste aversions when the head was the target for exposure rather than the abdomen. As with whole-body exposure, the aversion resulting from abdominal exposure became more severe as the radiation exposure was increased. On the other hand, increasing the exposure to the head beyond the threshold level made no difference in the severity of the aversion or in the rat's recovery to normal drinking. This is illustrated in Fig. 5.17. Here it can be seen

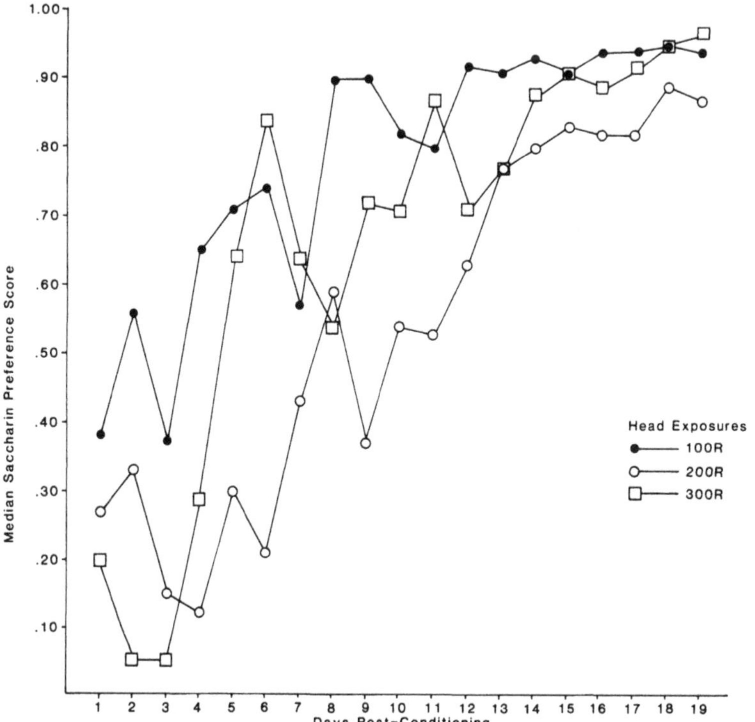

FIG. 5.17. Recovery from head-radiation-induced taste aversion; median saccharin preference scores are plotted as a function of post-conditioning test days for the exposure levels indicated.

that the 100, 200 and 300r exposures to the head resulted in comparable levels of aversion and comparable courses of recovery. Here again the implication is that some mechanism other than histamine production may be involved in the aversiveness of head-only exposure.

Further evidence for some facilitating role with head exposure was reported by Hunt et al. (1968). They found no saccharin aversion in the shielded partner at either 180r or 360r exposures when the irradiated partner of a parabiotic pair had the head shielded. This would make it appear that the radiation-induced taste aversion in the parabiotic rats resulted from causes which are different from those in the single rat treated with a pairing of saccharin and irradiation.

SUMMARY

In this chapter the suggestion has been made that taste aversion conditioning which has been induced in rats following irradiation may serve as a useful model for ascertaining the extent to which such conditioning could occur in human radiotherapy patients. We tested the assumption that some of the human dietary problems associated with cancer may be due to conditioned taste aversions inadvertently formed during the course of radiotherapy. The data presented here strongly suggest that such conditioning is possible in human patients. The data also suggest, however, that although learned taste aversions may contribute to the dietary problems, they do not seem to constitute a major part of the problem. The data also indicate that among the radiotherapy patients, those who are irradiated in the abdominal and pelvic region are more apt to show specific learned taste aversions than patients exposed in other body areas. It might be helpful to the radiotherapist and the oncologist to be aware that such aversions can be learned and that, potentially, steps can be taken to develop procedures to inhibit the radiation-induced conditioning process.

ACKNOWLEDGMENT

This research was supported by a grant (CA 22768) from the National Cancer Institute (DHEW). We would like to thank Alan Spector, Glee Hollander, and Denise Baker for help in the data collection and Denise Green, Anne Hightower and the TMRMC Radiotherapy Department staff for their assistance.

REFERENCES

Barker, L. M., & Smith, J. C. (1974). A comparison of taste aversions induced by radiation and lithium chloride in CS-US and US-CS paradigms. *Journal of Comparative and Physiology Psychology, 87,* 644–654.

Cairnie, A. B., & Leach, K. E. (1982). Dexamethasone: A potent blocker for radiation-induced taste aversion in rats. *Pharmacology Biochemistry and Behavior, 17,* 305–311.

Casarett, A. P. (1968). *Radiation Biology*. Englewood Cliffs, NJ: Prentice Hall.

Cooper, G., Kimeldorf, D. J., & McCarky, G. C. (1966). The effects of various gases within the nasal avitites of rats on the response of olfactory bulb neurons to x–radiation. *Radiation Research, 29*, 395–402.

DeWys, W. D., & Kisner, D. (1982). Principles of nutritional care of the cancer patient. In S. Carter, E. Glotstein, & R. B. Livingston (Eds.), *Principles of Cancer Treatment* (pp. 374–376). New York: McGraw-Hill.

Dinc, H. I., & Smith, J. C. (1966). Role of the olfactory bulbs in the detection of ionizing radiation by the rat. *Physiology and Behavior, 1*, 139–144.

Garcia, J., Ervin, F. R., & Koelling, R. A. (1967). Toxicity of serum from irradiated donors. *Nature, 213*, 682–683.

Garcia, J., & Hankins, W. G. (1977). On the origin of food aversion paradigms. In L. M. Barker, M. R. Best & M. Domjan (Eds.), *Learning Mechanisms in Food Selection*. Waco, TX: Baylor University Press.

Garcia, J., & Kimeldorf, D. J. (1960). Some factors which influence radiation-conditioned behavior of rats. *Radiation Research, 12*, 719–727.

Garcia, J., Kimeldorf, D. J., & Koelling, R. A. (1955). Conditioned aversion to saccharin resulting from exposure to gamma radiation. *Science, 122*, 157–158.

Garcia, J., & Koelling, R. A. (1967). A comparison of aversions induced by x–rays, toxins and drugs in the rat. *Radiation Research, 7*, 439–450.

Hunt, E. L., Carroll, H. W., & Kimeldorf, D. J. (1968). Effects of dose and partial body exposure on conditioning through a radiation-induced humoral factor. *Physiology and Behavior, 3*, 809–813.

Levy, C. J. (1975). *Histamine in taste aversions*. Paper presented at the 83rd annual convention of the American Psychological Association, Chicago, IL.

Levy, C. J., Carroll, M. E., Smith, J. C., & Hofer, K. G. (1974). Antihistamines block radiation-induced taste aversions. *Science, 186*, 1044–1046.

Levy, C. K., Ervin, F. R., & Garcia, J. (1970). Effect of serum from irradiated rats on gastrointestional function. *Nature, 225*, 463–464.

Peryam, D. R., & Pilgrim, F. J. (1957). Hedonic scale of measuring food preferences. *Food Technology, 11*(Suppl.), 4–14.

Reige, W. H. (1968). Possible olfactory transduction of radiation-induced aversion. *Psychonomic Science, 12*, 303–304.

Revusky, S., & Garcia, J. (1980). Learned associations over long delays. In G. W. Bowen & J. T. Spence (Eds.), *Psychology of Learning and Motivation: Advances in Research and Theory, Vol. 4* (pp. 1–84). New York: Academic Press.

Sessions, G. R. (1975). Histamine and radiation-induced taste aversion conditioning. *Science, 190*, 402–403.

Smith, J. C. (1971). Radiation: Its detection and its effects on taste preferences. In E. Stellar & J. M. Sprague (Eds.), *Progress in Physiological Psychology, Vol. 4*. New York: Academic Press.

Smith, J. C., Blumsack, J. T., Bilek, F. S., Spector, A. C., Hollander, G. R., & Baker, D. L. (1984). Radiation-induced taste aversion as a factor in cancer therapy. *Cancer Treatment Reports, 68*, 1219–1227.

Smith, J. C., & Roll, D. L. (1967). Trace conditioning with x–rays as an aversive stimulus. *Psychonomic Science, 9*, 11–12.

Smith, J. C., Hollander, G. R., & Spector, A. C. (1981). Taste aversions conditioned with partial body radiation exposures. *Physiology and Behavior, 27*, 903–913.

Spector, A. C., Smith, J. C., & Hollander, G. R. (1981). A comparison of dependent measures used to quantify radiation-induced taste aversion. *Physiology and Behavior, 27*, 887–901.

Spector, A. C., Smith, J. C., & Hollander, G. R. (1983). The effect of post-conditioning CS experience on recovery from radiation-induced taste aversion. *Physiology and Behavior, 30*, 647–649.

6 Learned Food Aversions: A Consequence of Cancer Chemotherapy

Ilene L. Bernstein
Mary M. Webster
University of Washington

Appetite and weight loss represent significant clinical problems affecting the well being of cancer patients and interfering with the delivery of effective treatment (Costa & Donaldson, 1979; Shils, 1979; Schein, Macdonald, Waters, & Haidak, 1975; Van Eys, 1979). The symptoms of many chemotherapy regimens can contribute directly to appetite and weight loss. In addition, these symptoms—principally nausea and vomiting (Borison & McCarthy, 1983; Laszlo, 1983)—are capable of functioning as unconditioned stimuli in the development of learned food aversions. In fact, some therapies used in the treatment of cancer (e.g., certain chemotherapeutic drugs; abdominal radiotherapy) are the same as those used to produce learned taste aversions in laboratory animals (Garcia, Hankins, & Rusiniak, 1974). Thus, at least part of the appetite suppression and altered food preferences in cancer patients may be an indirect or learned effect of the therapy and may be preventable by relatively simple intervention procedures which impede this learning.

In this chapter we review our early clinical research demonstrating that learned aversions to distinctively flavored foods can develop in children and adults receiving chemotherapy for cancer. We then describe a series of experiments with two animal models of chemotherapy-induced aversions which we have used to test potential intervention approaches. Finally we present evidence that cancer patients may also develop aversions to familiar diet items which they eat before gastrointestinal (GI) toxic chemotherapy and discuss methods for preventing these aversions.

LEARNED FOOD AVERSIONS IN PATIENTS RECEIVING CHEMOTHERAPY

Learned food aversions are aversions to specific foods (or tastes) which develop as a result of the association of those foods with unpleasant internal symptoms—such as nausea and vomiting (Garcia, Ervin, & Koelling, 1966; Garcia, Hankins, & Rusiniak, 1974). Most theorists consider taste aversion learning a variant of classical conditioning which evolved to enable animals to select nontoxic, nutritious substances for ingestion (Rozin & Kalat, 1971; Bolles, 1975). Special characteristics of this unusually potent form of learning have been widely documented in recent years (Riley & Clarke, 1977). Two of its most salient characteristics are (1) its rapid rate of acquisition (aversions frequently appear after a single conditioning trial) (Garcia, Hankins, & Rusiniak, 1974) and (2) its relative insensitivity to long delays (up to several hours) between the presentation of the conditioned stimulus (the taste of the food) and the onset of the unconditioned stimulus (the aversive internal symptoms) (Garcia, Ervin, & Koelling, 1966).

We thought it likely, given the compelling features of taste aversion learning, that humans exposed to pairings of foods and GI toxicity in the course of their cancer treatments would develop aversions to those foods. Interview studies (e.g., Garb & Stunkard, 1974) suggested that humans often develop profound distastes for foods that had been coincidentally associated with gastro-intestinal discomfort. The clinical setting provided an opportunity to examine taste aversion learning in humans experimentally. It was also important to determine whether learned food aversions were an inadvertent side effect of cancer chemotherapy, and whether ways could be devised to prevent them.

Our initial study examined learned taste aversions in pediatric cancer patients receiving chemotherapy (Bernstein, 1978). We asked whether children receiving drugs which were associated with nausea and vomiting would acquire aversions to a novel food consumed before their drug treatments. We used a novel food as our target stimulus because novel foods are apparently much more susceptible to aversion conditioning than are familiar foods (Revusky & Bedarf, 1967). The ''novel food'' target in this study was ''Mapletoff'' ice cream, chosen because children, even anxious and ''nondeprived'' children, are generally willing to eat ice cream. The novelty was introduced by using unusual flavoring, namely maple and black walnut flavor extracts.

Subjects were outpatients, between the ages of two and 16 years old, being treated at the Children's Orthopedic Hospital and Medical Center Hematology Clinic in Seattle. Patients scheduled to receive GI toxic chemotherapy (e.g., adriamycin, cyclophosphamide, cytosine arabinoside, nitrogen mustard) were randomly assigned to one of two groups: the Experimental Group (Group 1) which consumed Mapletoff ice cream shortly before their scheduled drug treatment, or the Drug Control Group (Group 2) which received similar drug treatments but no exposure to the ice cream. A Taste Control Group (Group 3) consisted of patients receiving chemotherapy not associated with GI symptoms (vincristine) or no drug treatment. Patients in this group consumed the same ice cream as the Experimental Group. Hence, this study consisted of an Experimental Group which received a single pairing of Mapletoff ice cream (CS) and symptoms of GI toxicity (US) and two Control Groups which were exposed only to the symptoms (US alone) or the ice cream (CS alone). Two or more weeks later, patients were tested for the development of aversions by being offered a choice between eating Mapletoff ice cream or playing with a game.

As shown in Table 6.1, only 21% of patients in the Experimental Group chose Mapletoff ice cream during the test session compared to 67% and 73% in the two Control Groups. The proportion of subjects selecting ice cream in Group 1 is significantly lower than in the Control Groups ($p < .001$). These results indicate that children will avoid eating a food which has previously been associated with GI toxic chemotherapy. The aversions were not caused by the GI toxic drug treatments alone, since patients in Group 2 were not averse to eating the ice cream. Nor was this particular ice cream flavor distasteful; patients who had eaten it before (Group 3) were willing to eat it again.

To evaluate the flavor specificity of these aversions, we later offered experimental and control patients a choice between two ice cream flavors, Mapletoff (the flavor paired with GI toxic therapy in the experimental group) and Hawaiian Delight (a novel, orange-pineapple ice cream). We asked the patients to taste both ice cream flavors, indicate which they preferred, and eat as much of each as they wished. Flavor preference and amount consumed were recorded. Preference for Mapletoff ice cream, whether measured by the amount consumed or the patients' stated preference, was significantly lower in the Experimental Group than in the Control Groups. Thus, aversions appear to be specific to the particular ice cream flavor presented during conditioning.

TABLE 6.1
Choice Made by Patients During Test Session[a]

	Number of Patients Selecting Ice Cream
Group 1 (Ice cream paired with GI toxicity)	3/14 (21%)
Group 2 (GI toxicity alone)	8/12 (67%)
Group 3 (Ice cream alone)	11/15 (73%)

[a]Reprinted from Bernstein, 1978, by permission. Copyright 1978 by AAAS.

Although finding taste aversion learning in human subjects was not entirely unexpected, there are some interesting features of these results. First, the aversions were acquired in a single conditioning trial even though lengthy delays were likely to have elapsed between the tasting of the ice cream and the experiencing of symptoms. (Symptoms may begin a few minutes to a few hours after drug administration.) Second, many of the patients had received a large number of prior drug treatments and most of them were old enough to understand that the cause of their symptoms of nausea and vomiting was their drug therapy and not Mapletoff ice cream. Because these factors would be expected to reduce aversion conditioning, the demonstration of significant aversions suggests that humans are relatively susceptible to taste aversion learning.

These studies were subsequently extended to an adult patient population (Bernstein & Webster, 1980). It was postulated that, because adults have a more complete understanding of the source of their drug symptoms, they may be less likely than children to acquire learned taste aversions. Seventy adult oncology patients were divided into Experimental and Control Groups based on their scheduled clinic treatment. Experimental subjects received chemotherapy likely to produce nausea and vomiting; control subjects received vincristine (no GI toxicity) or no drugs.

All the subjects were exposed to one of two distinctively flavored ice creams (Maple Nut or Hawaiian Delight) 15 to 60 minutes prior to drug treatment or check up. At a later clinic visit, subjects were tested for their flavor preferences in a two ice-cream choice test: They were asked to taste both ice cream flavors, indicate which they preferred, and eat as much of each as they wished. Statements of flavor preference and actual amounts consumed were recorded as in the previous experiment.

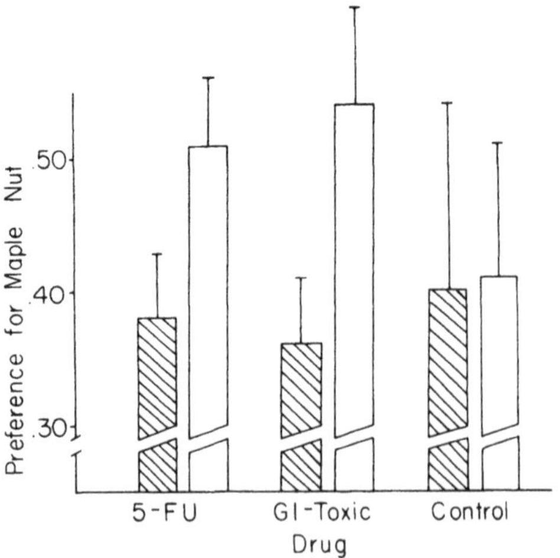

FIG. 6.1. Preference ratios for maple nut ice cream (+ SEM) based on actual ice cream consumption (g of maple nut consumed/ g of total ice cream consumed). Striped bars represent subjects preexposed to maple nut during conditioning; white bars represent subjects preexposed to Hawaiian delight. Preferences of experimental patients are presented separately depending on whether they received 5-fluorouracil (5-FU) or other "GI toxic drugs." Reprinted with permission from Bernstein & Webster (1980).

Preference scores, based on ice cream consumption during testing, are presented in Fig. 6.1. A lower preference for the particular flavor consumed prior to GI toxic drug treatment indicates the presence of a learned aversion to that flavor. Subjects in the Experimental Group who consumed Maple Nut ice cream during conditioning had a lower preference for that flavor than those who consumed Hawaiian Delight. This effect was not seen in the Control Group, where specific flavor exposure had no effect on preference. The aversions appear to be specific learned responses dependent on a single pairing of a flavor with an aversive drug treatment. Therefore, adults, like children (and numerous subhuman species), acquire learned taste aversions in a single trial. Apparently the cognitive development of adults, which enables them to understand the cause of their discomfort, does not override this conditioning.

ANIMAL MODELS OF THERAPY-INDUCED AVERSIONS

Since taste–aversion studies in the rat originally pointed us toward the existence of therapy-induced aversions in humans, it seemed particularly appropriate to turn to animal models of these aversions to understand more about the mechanisms involved and to test potential intervention approaches.

The vast majority of previous taste–aversion studies have employed deprived subjects and novel, flavored solutions. Therefore, our first task was to design a paradigm which would more closely model the clinical situation. It is obvious that a number of important differences exist between the eating habits of laboratory rats and human patients. Laboratory rats are typically raised from weaning on a single, complete food (e.g., commercial laboratory chow). Humans in our society, on the other hand, have a dazzling variety of foods available to them throughout life. Thus, differences in dietary variety and familiarity need to be considered in designing an appropriate rat model of therapy-induced aversions. Frankly, we have not tackled the "variety" issue yet, as the task of measuring intake of "supermarket foods" (e.g. Sclafani and Springer, 1976) discouraged us. We chose instead to provide a single, complete diet which was introduced prior to beginning a course of drug (cyclophosphamide) treatments. The aim was to provide a target food which was not totally novel, but also was not as familiar as laboratory chow (Bernstein, Vitiello & Sigmundi, 1980). Animals were preexposed to this diet (AIN diet; ICN, Cleveland, Ohio) for five days before receiving either four ip injections of cyclophosphamide (20 mg/kg; which is in the low range of dosages in clinical use) or 0.9% saline. Two recovery days elapsed between each injection with AIN diet continuously available ad lib throughout the 12 days. The acquisition of food aversions was evaluated in a 24-hr two food preference test, with a choice between AIN diet and a novel diet of comparable palatability. Drug-treated animals displayed significantly lower preferences than saline-treated controls for the AIN target diet, indicating that they had developed reliable aversions to the AIN diet (see Fig. 6.2). These findings are interesting because the animals were not deprived, and in fact had received five days of "safe" pre-exposure to the AIN diet prior to the first drug treatment. Furthermore the diet was present continuously during the 17-day experiment, rather than being presented only in temporal proximity to the drug treatments.

This treatment model was capable of producing significant diet aversions, allowing us to test a variety of intervention methods for reducing or eliminating the aversions. We rated the success of these interventions by the degree to which they reduced aversions to the AIN diet. The approaches evaluated were: (1) depriving animals of food for six hours before and after each drug treatment; (2) introducing a novel flavor in the animals' water around the time of each treatment; (3) exposing animals to a combination of food deprivation and novelly flavored water; and (4) replacing the animals' standard AIN diet with a novel food on treatment days. As can be seen in Fig. 6.3 only the introduction of a novel diet on treatment days was effective in preventing diet aversions. In spite of the fact that the animals in the Novel Diet group consumed very little of the novel food (and therefore would appear to be similar to the Deprivation group), aversions to the AIN diet were completely eliminated. Food deprivation and novel liquid interference stimuli did not reliably reduce the magnitude of AIN aversions. The lack of interference by flavored solutions was not due to a failure of these solutions to become conditioned aversive stimuli; strong aversions were acquired to the liquid flavor cues as well as to the target diet. These results suggest that exposure to a novel food interference stimulus might be effective in preventing or reducing learned food aversions to standard diet items in cancer patients receiving chemotherapy.

The study pointed to differences in the effectiveness of liquid and solid ingestibles as interference stimuli. A novel liquid failed to attenuate food aver-

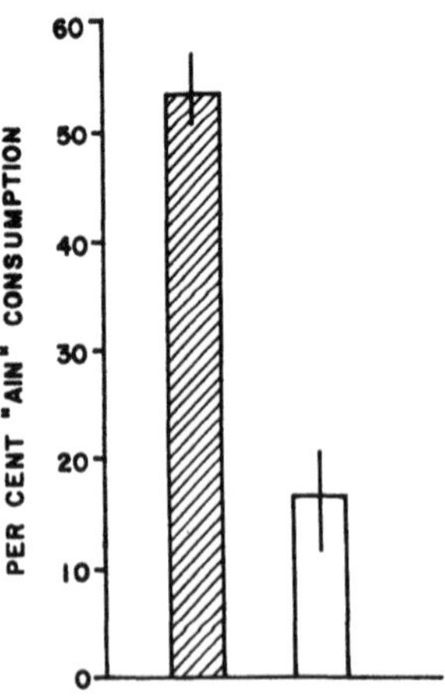

FIG. 6.2. Average preference (+ SE) for AIN meal in the 24-hr two-food choice test (AIN vs. chocolate chow). White bar: Drug-treated group; striped bar: Saline-treated controls. Based on data presented in Bernstein, Vitiello, & Sigmundi (1980).

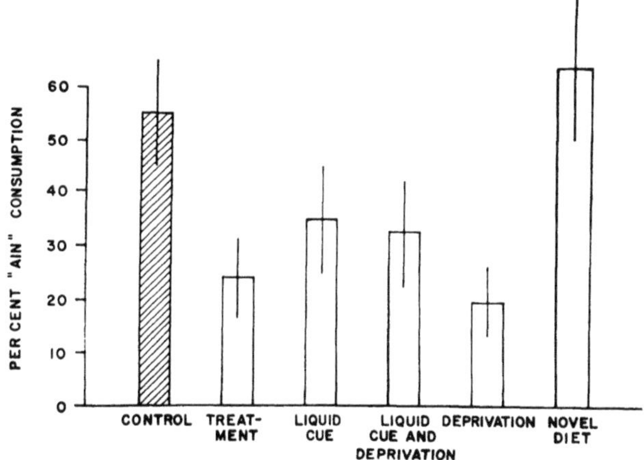

FIG. 6.3. Average preference (± SE) for AIN meal in the 24-hr two-food choice test (AIN meal vs. chocolate chow). Reprinted with permission from Bernstein, Vitiello, & Sigmundi (1980). Copyright 1980 by the American Psychological Association.

sions while a novel food completely blocked aversions to the target food. This observation led us to a series of studies designed to examine more closely the basis for the difference between liquids and foods in aversion conditioning (Bernstein, Goehler, & Bouton, 1983). These studies employed a somewhat more conventional taste–aversion paradigm, which consisted of exposing mildly deprived animals to novel foods and/or drinks during two-hour conditioning sessions. In all these studies animals were first trained to consume a daily meal of wet mash (tap water and Wayne Lab Blox) to ensure food and water ingestion during subsequent 2-hour conditioning sessions.

In the initial study animals received two conditioning sessions in which they were exposed either to (1) a novel food (AIN diet) alone; (2) a novel liquid (2% vinegar solution) alone; or (3) both the novel food and the novel liquid. All groups were then injected with cyclophosphamide (40 mg/kg). Aversions to the food and the liquid stimuli were evaluated in separate "single–choice" tests. We examined aversions to both the food and the liquid in order to determine whether aversions to one type of stimulus interfered with the development of aversions to the other. A total of six test trials for AIN and six test trials for vinegar solution were obtained for each subject. Comparisons of AIN consumption over the six test sessions (shown in Fig. 6.4) indicated that aversions to AIN diet were marked by little or no consumption of that diet during test sessions. This figure also shows that the presence of a novel liquid during food aversion conditioning did not interfere with the development of aversions to the target (AIN) diet. These findings are contrasted with the conditioning of liquid (vinegar) aversions (Fig. 6.5). Aversions to the vinegar solution are clearly evident. Furthermore,

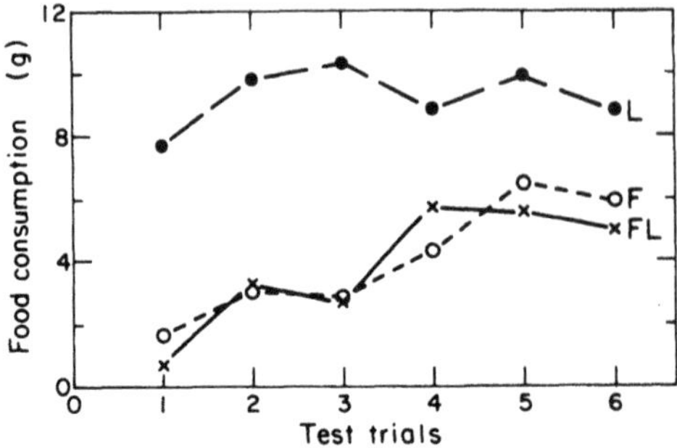

FIG. 6.4. Average consumption of AIN diet during six test sessions of groups conditioned with AIN alone (F), vinegar alone (L), or both AIN and vinegar (FL). Reprinted with permission from Bernstein, Goehler, & Bouton (1983).

aversion to the vinegar in the interference group was weaker than in the group exposed only to vinegar. Thus, although liquids did not interfere with the conditioning of foods, foods did interfere with the conditioning of liquids; moreover, the failure of vinegar to interfere with AIN aversions was not due to its failure to be noticed since significant aversions were conditioned to it as well as to AIN diet.

In the next study we examined whether a second food would be effective in interfering with the conditioning of the target diet in this "meal feeding" paradigm. Animals were exposed to either one novel food (AIN) or two novel foods (AIN and C-21) (Bernstein et al., 1983) during two conditioning sessions. A control group received familiar wet mash (as during meal training). Daily test sessions began two days after the second drug injections and continued for 23 days.

Consumption of the target AIN diet over 23 test sessions is depicted in Fig. 6.6. An aversion to AIN is evident when the two groups exposed to novel food(s) during conditioning are compared to controls; however, there is no evidence that the group exposed to two foods developed milder aversions to AIN than the

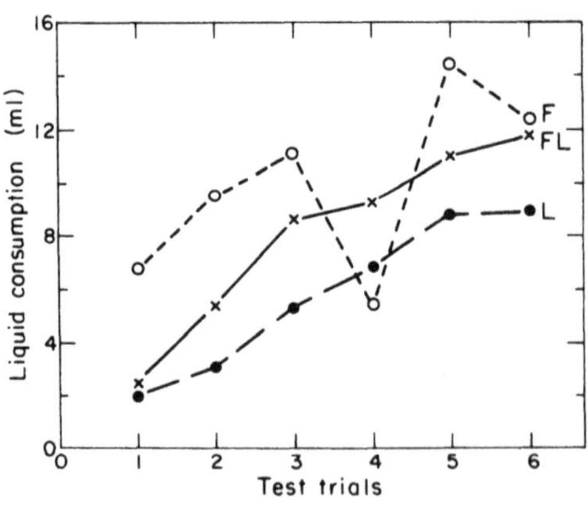

FIG 6.5. Average consumption of vinegar solution during six test sessions of groups conditioned with vinegar alone (L), AIN alone (F), or both AIN and vinegar (FL). Reprinted with permission from Bernstein, Goehler, & Bouton (1983).

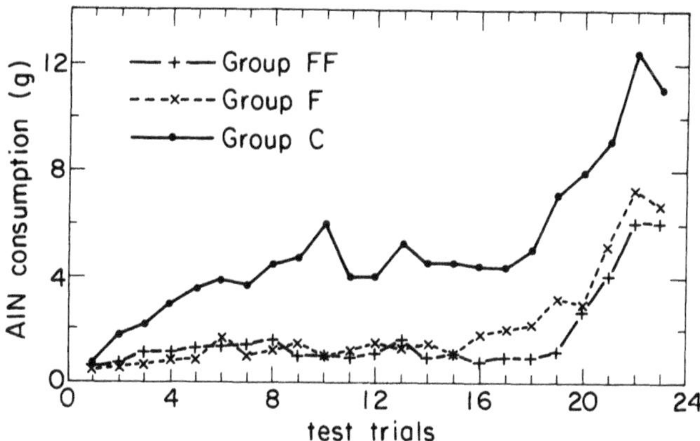

FIG. 6.6. Average consumption of AIN diet over test trials of groups conditioned with AIN alone (F), AIN and C-21 (FF), or wet mash (Controls).

group exposed to AIN alone. Both groups show profound and long lasting aversions to AIN diet. Thus, in this paradigm, novel foods as well as novel liquids failed to interfere with aversions to a novel target diet. This differs from our previous interference studies where a novel food but not a novel liquid interfered with target diet aversions (Bernstein et al., 1980). However, both the target and interfering food in the present study were novel, and both had a close temporal relation to the drug injections. Furthermore, a higher dose of cyclophosphamide was used. Apparently, under these conditions, target foods are relatively resistant to interference produced by other foods as well as liquids.

These findings, as well as those of related studies done in our lab, point to unusual properties of foods as targets for aversions. Novel foods, unlike novel drinks, are very resistant to interference effects. A number of differences between our ''food'' stimuli and our ''drink'' stimuli could have contributed to the robustness of food aversions. Among them are the flavor intensity and nutrient density of foods relative to drinks. Parametric differences along a continuum like ''flavor intensity'' may be important determinants of these food–liquid differences. However, while it may be convenient to think of foods and liquids as lying along a single intensity continuum, we doubt that such a continuum exists in the real world. We believe that most foods are simply much more potent targets for aversion conditioning than most drinks. In fact it is tempting to suggest that taste aversion learning directed at dilute solutions reflects only a fraction of the potential potency observed when such learning is directed at a target food.

Having made a rather strong statement regarding interference with food aversions, we must add some important qualifications. The findings of the previous studies were interpreted as reflecting properties of the foods, or the CS. Another aspect of those experiments may have played a role in the resistance of food aversions to interference—namely the intensity of the conditioned aversions. It is important to determine whether interference with food aversions is more likely to be seen when the intensity of conditioned aversions is reduced. Two ways to accomplish this, while still using the same food target, are to reduce the dose of the drug or reduce the number of conditioning trials. Two recent studies in our laboratory examined this using the "meal feeding" paradigm to compare aversions to a target food when that food was conditioned alone or in combination with another food (Fenner & Bernstein, 1984). In the first study our only modification was to use one rather than two conditioning trials. In the second study the modification involved using a lower cyclophosphamide dose (20 mg/kg rather than 40 mg/kg). In both of these studies we found that the presence of a second food *did* interfere with the conditioning of aversions to the target food. In other words when the strength of aversion conditioning was reduced by reducing the magnitude of the US or reducing the number of training trials, a target food was no longer immune to interference by another food.

There is probably not a one-to-one correspondence between the various manipulations employed in these animal studies and the problem of designing effective clinical interventions. Nevertheless, it is useful to be aware of the numerous variables which can influence the potency of food aversion conditioning and its resistance to interference.

LEARNED AVERSIONS TO FAMILIAR FOODS

We now turn to the question of whether aversions affect patients' preference for familiar foods in their routine diets, and not just novel target foods (Bernstein, Webster, & Bernstein, 1982). This study used diet inventories or questionnaires to assess changes in food preferences and food choices as a result of GI toxic chemotherapy. Eighty-four pediatric patients completed diet inventories during an initial treatment session and again at a subsequent evaluation session at least a week later. These forms were completed at the same time that subjects were participating in the previously described "ice cream" study. Children (with the help of their parents) listed their favorite foods, foods they were reluctant to eat, and typical breakfast, lunch and dinner menus. During the initial session, they also indicated specific food items they had consumed in the four to five hour period before coming to the clinic. Patients receiving GI toxic chemotherapy composed the Experimental Group and the specific foods they had eaten before their drug therapy were considered the targets for the formation of aversions. To assess aversions the two questionnaires from each patient were compared and scored by a rater blind to the group membership of subjects; an aversion was scored when a specific food eaten before therapy was no longer preferred, became actively disliked, or was no longer listed in usual menus. Patients were classified as either showing an aversion or not. We determined the number of patients whose inventories showed at least one such aversion. Patients receiving vincristine or no drug provided a Control Group which allowed us to compare inventory changes in the Experimental Group to a comparable patient population not currently receiving GI toxic therapy. Control Group changes from Session 1 to Session 2 provide an estimate of the rate such changes occur due to chance, forgetting or some other factor.

Multiple regression analysis was performed to indicate which variables best predicted the incidence of aversions. Results of this analysis showed that the number of food items consumed before therapy made the greatest contribution to the variance in incidence of aversions. We then controlled for the number of "pretherapy items" in the analysis and classified patients in the Experimental Group with regard to whether they had consumed Mapletoff ice cream before treatment (Group 1) or not (Group 2). We then compared each of these Experimental Groups to the Control Group. We found that GI toxic drug treatment was significantly associated with the incidence of aversions in Group 2, where those nausea symptoms were experienced without ice cream exposure (See Table 2). Incidence of aversions in Group 1 was intermediate between controls (Group 3) and Group 2 and did not differ significantly from either. Thus Group 1 patients exposed to a novel taste (Mapletoff ice cream) before treatments did not show a significantly higher incidence of aversions than controls. These patients were randomly selected from those scheduled for GI toxic therapy, and in fact reported somewhat more severe drug symptoms (nausea, vomiting) than patients not exposed to ice cream. The observation that drug treatment was significantly associated with the formation of diet aversions only in the group not exposed to ice cream suggests that the ice cream may have blocked the development of

TABLE 6.2
Aversions to Foods in the Diet[b]

	No. of Patients[a] Showing Aversions
Group 1	
GI toxic drugs/ice cream	14/25 (56%)
Group 2	
GI toxic drugs/no ice cream	16/23 (70%)
Group 3	
Controls	11/31 (36%)

[a]Difference between two proportions: Groups 1 and 2 (combined) versus Group 3 =$p<0.02$.
[b]Reprinted from Bernstein, Webster, and Bernstein, 1982, by permission.

aversions to foods in the diet. It should be noted that this study was not designed to examine interference effects, but was rather a serendipitous result of looking at diet aversions in the same patients that had been in the "ice cream study". The findings are suggestive of an interference effect which clearly needs to be examined further. However, these observations are consistent with some of the results of our animal studies; namely that a novel taste presented in association with toxic drug treatment can interfere with aversions to a target food. Perhaps deliberate exposure in the clinic to novel, "scapegoat" tastes prior to chemotherapy treatments would protect normal diet items from becoming the targets for learned food aversions. A study explicitly designed to test this possibility is currently in progress. One problem we anticipate is that conditioning of the scapegoat stimulus may occur, such that with repeated trials patients will become reluctant to consume it. Therefore, it may be necessary to change the scapegoat frequently in order for this procedure to be useful with patients receiving repeated chemotherapy trials.

The prevalence of aversions to familiar diet items in our pediatric population is somewhat surprising in view of the emphasis placed on stimulus novelty in the taste aversion literature. Possible explanations of our findings include the following: (1) Foods appear to be far more potent stimuli for taste aversion conditioning than are flavored solutions, and conclusions based largely on studies using flavored solutions may not apply. (2) If children tend to consume particular foods repeatedly for breakfast or lunch, when they receive multiple chemotherapy treatments, one or more of those foods may receive multiple conditioning trials. Repeated trials increase the likelihood of aversions to familiar foods (Elkins, 1974). (3) Familiar foods may taste "novel" to cancer patients because cancer and cancer therapy can induce changes in taste bud function (Conger, 1973; DeWys, 1974).

SUMMARY AND FUTURE DIRECTIONS

In this chapter we reviewed our clinical studies indicating that learned taste aversions can arise in pediatric and adult cancer patients as a consequence of consuming a novel target food before receiving GI toxic chemotherapy. We also described results of a questionnaire study which suggested that aversions may arise to familiar items in patients' routine diets as a result of their association with chemotherapy. In a series of animal studies which modelled certain features of the clinical situation, we tested a variety of intervention methods for reducing or eliminating learned food aversions. Presentation of a novel liquid before drug treatments failed to attenuate food aversions. A novel food, on the other hand, was a more effective interference stimulus than a novel liquid. However, uder certain conditions, target foods were found to be quite resistant to interference produced either by other foods or by novel liquids. Interference with food aversions was more likely to occur when the intensity of conditioned aversions was reduced. These animal studies provide information about the variables which can potentially influence the success of clinical intervention approaches.

Examination of food aversions in clinic patients provided additional clues to possible clinical interventions. For example, the consumption of a novel "scapegoat" taste may provide some protection against the development of aversions to familiar foods in patients' routine diets. We have recently begun a clinical study to evaluate the effectiveness of a "scapegoat" stimulus in preventing diet aversions.

ACKNOWLEDGMENT

This research was supported by NIH Grant RO1-CA26419.

Requests for reprints should be sent to Ilene L. Bernstein, Department of Psychology, NI-25, University of Washington, Seattle, Washington 98195.

REFERENCES

Bernstein, I. L. (1978). Learned taste aversions in children receiving chemotherapy. *Science, 200,* 1302–1303.

Bernstein, I. L., Goehler, L. E., & Bouton, M. E. (1983). Relative potency of foods and drinks as targets in aversion conditioning. *Behavioral and Neural Biology, 37,* 134–148.

Bernstein, I. L., Vitiello, M. V., & Sigmundi, R. A. (1980). Effects of interference stimuli on the acquisition of learned aversions to foods in the rat. *Journal of Comparative and Physiological Psychology, 94,* 921–931.

Bernstein, I. L., & Webster, M. M. (1980). Learned taste aversions in humans. *Physiology and Behavior, 25,* 363–366.

Bernstein, I. L., Webster, M. M., & Bernstein, I. D. (1982). Food aversions in children receiving chemotherapy for cancer. *Cancer, 50,* 2961–2963.

Bolles, R. C. (1975). *Learning theory.* New York: Holt, Rinehart and Winston.

Borison, H. L., & McCarthy, L. E. (1983). Neuropharmacology of chemotherapy-induced emesis. *Drugs, 25* (Suppl. 1), 8–17.

Conger, A. D. (1973). Loss and recovery of taste acuity in patients irradiated to the oral cavity. *Radiation Research, 53,* 338–347.

Costa, G., & Donaldson, S. S. (1979). Effects of cancer and cancer treatment on the nutrition of the host. *New England Journal of Medicine, 300,* 1471.

DeWys, W. D. (1974). Abnormalities of taste as a remote effect of a neoplasm. *Annals of the New York Academy of Science, 230,* 427–434.

Elkins, R. L. (1974). Conditioned flavor aversions to familiar tap water in rats: An adjustment with implications for aversion therapy treatment of alcoholism and obesity. *Journal of Abnormal Psychology, 83,* 4, 411–417.

Fenner, D. P., & Bernstein, I. L. (1984). Interference in food aversion conditioning by reducing drug dose or conditioning trials. *Behavioral and Neural Biology, 40,* 114–118.

Garb, J. L., & Stunkard, A. J. (1974). Taste aversions in man. *American Journal of Psychiatry, 131,* 1204–1207.

Garcia, J., Ervin, F. R., & Koelling, R. A. (1966). Learning with prolonged delay of reinforcement. *Psychonomic Science, 5,* 121–122.

Garcia, J., Hankins, W. G., & Rusiniak, K. W. (1974). Behavioral regulation of the milieu interne in man and rat. *Science, 185,* 824–831.

Laszlo, J. (1983). Nausea and vomiting as major complications of cancer chemotherapy. *Drugs, 25* (Suppl. 1), 1–7.

Revusky, S. H., & Bedarf, E. W. (1967). Association of illness with prior ingestion of novel foods. *Science, 155,* 219–220.

Riley, A. L., & Clarke, C. M. (1977). Conditioned taste aversions: A bibliography. In L. M. Barker, M. R. Best, & M. Domjan (Eds.), *Learning Mechanisms in Food Selection.* Waco, TX.: Baylor University Press.

Rozin, P., & Kalat, J. W. (1971). Specific hungers and poison avoidance as adaptive specializations of learning. *Psychological Review, 78,* 459–486.

Schein, P. S., Macdonald, J. S., Waters, C., & Haidak, D. (1975). Nutritional complications of cancer and its treatment. *Seminars of Oncology, 2,* 337–347.

Sclafani, A., & Springer, D. (1976). Dietary obesity in adult rats: Similarities to hypothalamic and human obesity syndromes. *Physiology and Behavior, 17,* 461–471.

Shils, M. E. (1979). Nutritional problems induced by cancer. *Medical Clinics of North America, 63,* 1009–1025.

Van Eys, J. (1979). Malnutrition in children with cancer. *Cancer, 43,* 2030–2035.

7 Aversive Conditioning and Cancer Chemotherapy

William H. Redd
University of Illinois

Thomas G. Burish
Vanderbilt University

Michael A. Andrykowski
University of Illinois

Cytotoxic chemotherapy is routinely used in the treatment of cancer. Either alone or in combination with surgery and/or radiation, chemotherapy typically involves repeated infusions of highly toxic drugs which can produce severe side effects. These include decreased immunity to disease, hair loss, fatigue, changes in body weight, sterility, nausea, and emesis (Golden, 1975). Unfortunately, such effects often become more noxious and debilitating with repeated infusions (Love, Nerenz, & Leventhal, 1982). During the protracted course of treatment some patients develop what appear to be nonpharmacological side effects. After two or three infusions these patients may become nauseated and/or vomit *before* the cytotoxic drugs would be expected to produce such effects. Patients frequently begin vomiting while the drugs are being injected or while the nurse cleans the skin with alcohol in preparation for the infusion. There are patients who feel nauseated as they approach the hospital for treatment; others report that even talking about chemotherapy makes them nauseated.

The purpose of this chapter is to discuss the development of anticipatory and nonpharmacological side effects associated with cancer chemotherapy. The discussion first considers the prevalence of such side effects and then focuses on the mechanisms that may underlie their development. Attention is also devoted to factors that might predispose individuals to develop these aversion reactions.

PREVALENCE OF ANTICIPATORY SIDE EFFECTS

Although considerable research effort has been directed toward determining the prevalence of anticipatory reactions in patients, precise data are not available. Fourteen separate studies have been reported since 1980 (Cohen, Sheehan, Ruckdeschel, & Blanchard, 1982; Coons, 1982; Fetting, Wilcox, Iwata, Criswell, Bosmajian, & Sheidler, 1983; Love, Nerenz, & Leventhal, 1982; Morrow, 1982; Morrow, Arsineau, Asbury, Bennett, & Boros, 1982; Nerenz, Leventhal, & Love, 1982; Nerenz, Leventhal, Love, Coons, & Ringler, 1982; Nesse, Carli, Curtis, & Kleinman, 1980; Nicholas, 1982; Penta, Poster, Bruno, & Jacobs, 1983; Schulz, 1980; Scogna & Smalley, 1979; Wilcox, Fetting, Netteschim, & Abeloff, 1982) and estimates of the numbers of patients who develop such symptoms vary greatly. For example, Schulz (1980) collected questionnaire data from 68 chemotherapy patients who had received treatment for at least two months and found that 21 patients (31%) reported experiencing nausea and/or emesis prior to or during chemotherapy infusions. On the other hand, Nesse et al. (1980) reported that eight of the 18 (44%) lymphoma patients interviewed experienced mild to severe anticipatory nausea/emesis. In interviews with 41 breast cancer patients, Scogna and Smalley (1979) found that 27% of the patients reported anticipatory nausea/emesis.

These discrepancies in reported prevalence appear to reflect differences in how the studies were conducted. Through the wisdom of hindsight, we can identify three methodological problems contributing to the lack of consistent findings. The first concerns the criteria used to establish the presence of anticipatory side effects. Some investigators have included in their pool of subjects individuals experiencing *either* anticipatory nausea or anticipatory vomiting, while others have studied only those patients who experience *both* reactions. The effect that this difference has on reported prevalence is illustrated in Morrow et al.'s (1982) comprehensive assessment of behavioral side effects of chemotherapy. When the presence of anticipatory vomiting was needed to meet the criterion, only 9% of their sample of chemotherapy patients could be identified as experiencing anticipatory side effects; however, when anticipatory nausea was the sole criterion, 24% of the sample were included.

The second problem involves the scheduling of data collection; i.e., the point during the course of repeated chemotherapy treatments at which patients were interviewed and relevant information was obtained. The problem stems from the fact that the probability that patients will experience anticipatory side effects generally increases with repeated exposures to chemotherapy and its posttreatment side effects (Nerenz, Leventhal, Love, Coons, & Ringler, 1982). Thus, if assessments of pretreatment nausea and emesis were conducted relatively early during the course of treatment, generally lower prevalence rates would be expected. Likewise, if assessments were carried out later, higher rates would be more likely. Unfortunately, no standardized data collection schedule has been established in the research published to date. Some investigators have reported data obtained after the first or second cycle of chemotherapy, while others have presented data obtained after the last cycle. Moreover, when researchers have assessed anticipatory side effects late in the course of treatments, they have generally not determined when patients first experienced such reactions.

The third problem concerns the fact that prevalence data have not been systematically obtained for particular drug protocols. Since protocols vary in their emeticity, and because drugs with greater emeticity (such as cisplatin) are associated with greater pretreatment side effects, it is necessary to specify prevalence rates for particular protocols. For example, Nerenz, Leventhal, Love, Coons, & Ringler (1982) reported that 65% of their patients receiving cisplatin exhibited anticipatory side effects, whereas only 15% of patients receiving the less emetic CMF protocol (cytoxan, methotrexate and 5-FU) developed anticipatory reactions. Unfortunately, some investigators have reported prevalence rates without specifying the drug protocol(s) patients were receiving or have combined data for different protocols without determining the contribution of each.

Because of these methodological problems it is impossible to determine from the available data the exact prevalence rates of anticipatory side effects. Nonetheless, it is clear that anticipatory side effects do affect a considerable number of patients; even a conservative overall figure would put the prevalence rate at 25% or more. However, determination of the prevalence of anticipatory reactions to chemotherapy must be pursued with greater sophistication than is provided by overall prevalence estimates. What is needed is information regarding the prevalence of anticipatory nausea, vomiting, anxiety, etc. for particular drug protocols, for identified groups of patients, reassessed at regular intervals during the course of chemotherapy. Such research will allow us to make clinically meaningful predictions regarding the development of anticipatory reactions and will contribute to our theoretical understanding of aversive conditioning.

MECHANISMS UNDERLYING THE DEVELOPMENT OF ANTICIPATORY NAUSEA/EMESIS

Research on anticipatory side effects of chemotherapy has generally focused on describing the parameters of the phenomenon and on methods of controlling or ameliorating it. Little research has investigated mechanisms underlying the development of these side effects. Our understanding of possible mechanisms comes from indirect evidence and theoretical speculation. At least five hypotheses have been offered to explain these symptoms (Burish & Carey, 1984). These explanations view anticipatory nausea/emesis as the result of one of the following: (1) underlying psychological readjustment problems associated with life-threatening illness; (2) severe anxiety experienced immediately before treatment; (3) physiological changes associated with advanced disease; (4) operant conditioning; or (5) respondent conditioning.

Psychological Readjustment Problems

Based on clinical observation Chang (1981) has hypothesized that anticipatory nausea and vomiting "may be surfacing manifestations of underlying psychological readjustment problems associated with life-threatening illness" (p. 707). He suggested further that nonpharmacological side effects develop in those patients who cannot fully accept the diagnosis of cancer and the treatment it requires. Consequently, these patients become angry, anxious, and frustrated. Because they have no target for their negative feelings, they redirect these emotional reactions toward the chemotherapy treatment by exhibiting "psychological" side effects. Unfortunately, Chang provided no theoretical rationale or empirical support for his thesis. Without substantive data, Chang's hypotheses can only be viewed as interesting speculations.

Anxiety

Another possibility is that anticipatory nausea and emesis result from anxiety which increases as the time for scheduled chemotherapy draws near. Such anxiety-produced nausea/emesis has been observed in athletes immediately before an important competitive event (Katahn, 1967) and in some individuals anticipating other stressors (e.g., Swanson, Swenson, Huizenga, & Melson, 1976). Although no direct support for this hypothesis has been generated in the research on chemotherapy side effects, correlations between anxiety experienced during treatment and anticipatory nausea/emesis have been found in two separate studies (Love, Nerenz, & Leventhal, 1982; Nerenz, Leventhal, & Love, 1982). Patients with anticipatory nausea/emesis reported higher levels of anxiety than patients who did not experience such side effects. Patients who had anticipatory symptoms also experienced greater emotional distress associated with treatment. Of course reported anxiety and distress may have resulted from, rather than have caused, anticipatory side effects.

In addition to the uncertainty of the causal direction of the anxiety-nausea relationship, other lines of reasoning and some available data reduce our confidence in the explanatory power of the hypothesis. If heightened anxiety were the cause of anticipatory nausea/emesis, one might expect that patients who display these reactions would also experience nausea and emesis in other stressful situations. In light of the extensive evidence for specificity across individuals in their physiological responses to anxiety-producing situations and other types of stressors (Lacey, 1967), individuals who display anticipatory nausea and/or vomiting in the chemotherapy situation might also be expected to have histories of anxiety-induced nausea/emesis in other situations. However, a careful review of patients' histories revealed that none of the 55 patients showing anticipatory symptoms in the Morrow (1982) or in the Nesse et al. (1980) studies had ever vomited or reported feeling nauseated in stressful situations. Of course, it is possible that chemotherapy represented the most stressful life experience for these patients and, therefore, was the only situation that evoked nausea/emesis.

While such a counter explanation is plausible, an examination of pediatric patients' reactions to bone marrow aspiration reveals patterns of responding that are inconsistent with the anxiety hypothesis. Bone marrow aspiration is an extremely painful procedure and can be as stressful as chemotherapy. Indeed, the vast majority of children actively resist the procedure, and it is not unusual for two or three nurses to be called to restrain a child while the physician completes the procedure. Katz, Kellerman, and Seigel (1980) reported that 97% of the children they studied exhibited severe anxiety reactions before and during bone marrow aspiration, yet less than 2% of the children became nauseated or vomited in anticipation of the procedure. In our clinical work, we have treated children who vomited before scheduled chemotherapy infusions, yet did not experience nausea or emesis before bone marrow aspirations, despite the fact that they violently resisted bone marrow aspirations.

Although neither line of evidence can be considered as conclusive, it appears unlikely that anxiety is the sole factor causing anticipatory symptoms associated with chemotherapy.

Physiological Mechanisms

It has been hypothesized that anticipatory symptoms may "be produced by brain metastasis or local cancer involvement of the gastrointestinal tract" (Chang, 1981, p. 707). While this explanation may be true for a few patients, it seems unlikely that it accounts for the development of anticipatory symptoms in most patients. For example, when Morrow (1982) screened 47 patients with anticipatory nausea for brain metastases and gastrointestinal tumors that might cause nausea or vomiting, he found that none of the patients evidenced brain metastases or gastrointestinal tumors.

Another problem with this explanation is that if brain metastases were the contributing factor, then patients with anticipatory nausea/emesis should also display severe nausea across diverse situations. They do not; in all of the reported cases, profuse nausea/emesis occurred only in response to specific stimuli. Thus, it seems clear that the physiological explanation for non-pharmacological side effects of chemotherapy does not adequately account for the phenomenon.

Operant Conditioning

It is conceivable that anticipatory symptoms could represent operant behaviors under the control of contingencies of social reinforcement. Like the operant pain behaviors identified by Fordyce (1973), anticipatory side effects could serve as a means of evoking greater care-giving from others and of escaping undesired activities and responsibilities. Research has shown that individuals can exercise instrumental control over physiological responses such as heart rate, galvanic skin response, vasodilation, etc., that previously were believed not to be subject to voluntary control (e.g., Katkin, 1976). There are also reports in the literature of the modification of maladaptive physiological responses through the withdrawal of contingencies of social reinforcement (Ingersoll & Curry, 1977). However, none of the research on the development and behavioral control of anticipatory side effects has addressed this possibility. However, from our clinical observation and experience, it would appear that nurses and physicians in oncology settings do not specifically "reward" the display of anticipatory nausea/emesis. Medical staff generally view such symptoms as annoyances that make their duties more difficult. Although family members are typically sympathetic, they often share the patient's embarrassment surrounding his or her uncontrolled vomiting. In some instances patients are even chastised for their anticipatory symptoms. We once overheard a patient ridiculing another, saying: "Why are you throwing up before you even get the drugs? That's silly; it's all in your head." If operant mechanisms are involved, they would seem to involve most often the punishment of anticipatory reactions rather than their positive reinforcement.

Respondent Conditioning

The conceptualization of the development of anticipatory side effects as the result of respondent conditioning has received the widest acceptance among researchers in the area (Burish & Lyles, 1979; Katz, 1982; Morrow, 1982; Nesse et al., 1980; Redd & Andresen, 1981; Schulz, 1980). Through repeated pairings of chemotherapy and its pharmacologic side effects, previously neutral stimuli (e.g., the sights, sounds and odors of the treatment setting) can become potent elicitors of nausea and/or vomiting. The patient's acquired response to clinic stimuli is similar in form and intensity to the nausea and vomiting induced by the drugs used in chemotherapy. Thus, it is argued, stimuli in the treatment environment function as conditioned stimuli eliciting the conditioned response(s) (e.g., nausea and/or emesis).

Evidence supporting the respondent conditioning hypothesis is drawn from several sources: (1) early laboratory research on the effects of apomorphine injections on dogs (Pavlov, 1927); (2) research on taste aversion in animals (Robertson & Garcia, this volume); (3) experimental work on conditioned food aversion in chemotherapy patients (Bernstein & Webster, this volume); and (4) clinical findings on inadvertent aversive conditioning following chemotherapy infusions (Kutz, Borysenko, Come, & Benson, 1980; Morrow et al., 1982; Redd & Andresen, 1981). Each of these lines of evidence is examined below.

Pavlov (1927) noticed that, after repeated laboratory injections of the emetic drug apomorphine in dogs, the animals acquired a conditioned vomiting response to stimuli associated with the injections. After 5 or 6 days of exposure to apomorphine injections, the dogs would salivate and vomit in response to the sight of the syringe, the preparation of the skin for the injection and the sound of the tone that had been paired with the initial vomiting responses. In the most striking cases, dogs would display these symptoms at the mere sight of the investigator who had repeatedly administered the injections. Similar observations have also been reported by Collins and Tatum (1925). These results clearly show that under laboratory conditions emesis can develop as a conditioned response to external stimuli that regularly preceded the injection of an emesis-producing drug.

Additional support for the contention that anticipatory nausea/emesis can be a classically conditioned response comes from the apparent similarity of the development of these responses to the development of taste aversions. The acquisition of taste aversions in laboratory rats was originally demonstrated by Garcia and his colleagues (Garcia, Kimeldorf, & Koelling, 1955). Rats who drank a saccharin solution and who later became ill from exposure to gamma irradiation developed a strong aversion to the saccharin taste. This aversion was evidenced by subsequent avoidance of the previously preferred saccharin solution when the animal was given the opportunity to drink either water or the saccharin solution. Since this initial work an extensive experimental literature (see Robertson & Garcia, this volume; Riley & Clarke, 1977) has arisen, demonstrating that a variety of experimental animals will develop strong aversions to the taste of food that has been associated with illness. It is assumed, though not proven, that the animals would display "illness reactions" (i.e., retching, gagging, etc.) if they were *not* given the opportunity to avoid the stimulus and were forced to ingest the food. The development of such taste aversions has conventionally been accounted for in terms of a classical conditioning paradigm, with the taste of the food ingested viewed as the conditioned stimulus and the illness as the unconditioned response (Garcia, McGowan, & Green, 1972).

Obvious ethical considerations have prevented extensive experimental research on taste aversion in humans. However, survey research by Garb and Strunkard (1974) is relevant to our understanding of the development of chemotherapy-induced aversions and its similarity to taste aversion. They surveyed 696 people using a self-report questionnaire and found that 38% of their sample reported the presence of a specific food aversion at some point in their lives. In addition, 87% of the respondents who reported such aversions indicated that the aversion developed after they had become ill following consumption of that specific food item and that the aversion developed to the taste of the food. In general, it was found that the conditions and parameters under which these naturally occurring aversions developed were virtually identical to those of the traditional experimental food aversion paradigm.

Bernstein and her colleagues (see Bernstein & Webster, this volume) have attempted to experimentally induce taste aversions in human subjects, both children and adults. What is most significant about this research is that all of their subjects were cancer patients receiving chemotherapy. In these studies patients ate a novel flavor of ice cream (Mapletoff—maple and black walnut) 15 to 60 minutes prior to receiving their regularly scheduled chemotherapy treatment. The development of an aversion to the Mapletoff ice cream was assessed at a subsequent clinic visit, ranging from 2 to 16 weeks later. Patients who had Mapletoff ice cream paired with the illness resulting from chemotherapy ate significantly less of the Mapletoff at the later testing session than did control patients. Bernstein's research effectively demonstrates that chemotherapy-induced nausea and vomiting can function as an unconditioned stimulus in a traditional aversion learning paradigm; it also shows that such learning can occur despite the patient's knowledge that the particular food consumed was not the cause of the illness. Thus, cognitive factors appear to have little ability to override or prevent the development of taste aversions in humans.

Perhaps the clearest examples of classically conditioned nausea in humans come from clinical reports of patients' responses to stimuli repeatedly paired with their postchemotherapy nausea and emesis (Kutz et al., 1980; Morrow et al., 1982; Redd & Andresen, 1981). In preliminary analysis of the use of relaxation and distraction to control postchemotherapy nausea, Redd and Andresen enlisted the cooperation of six female patients being treated with cisplatin for ovarian cancer. One method used to reduce some of the unpleasant side effects of cisplatin is to give the patients high dosages of chlorpromazine (Thorazine) to sedate them and make it easier for them to "sleep through" the nausea. (This method is only partially effective and is far from popular with physicians and patients since chlorpromazine has its own unpleasant side effects.) Patients in this research were initially trained by a therapist in the use of self-hypnosis and then given an audiotape recording of one of their training sessions to use for practice and during subsequent posttreatment periods. The response was uniform: the hypnosis made them more comfortable and less nauseated, and the patients said they preferred using hypnosis to receiving chlorpromazine. Although hypnosis did not actually reduce emesis (as measured by volume produced), the patients said that they wanted to continue to use hypnosis. Because the patients used the tapes immediately following subsequent chemotherapy infusions, an interesting pattern of responding emerged. The patients began complaining that the sound of the therapist's voice made them nauseated. Although none of the patients actually vomited in response to the therapist's voice, they reported that the therapist's voice had become aversive. They stated that even talking to the therapist on the telephone made them slightly nauseated, and they admitted preferring not to communicate by phone. All six of the subjects had the same experience. Of course, the patients were free to stop using the tape, and four of the six did so. Interestingly, these four reported that they planned to continue to use self-hypnosis, but without the tape. These responses suggest that the strong effect of the drug outweighed the effect of the hypnosis and the tape, similar to what occurs with other stimuli associated with chemotherapy. The therapist's voice became a conditioned stimulus, eliciting nausea.

A similar phenomenon has been reported by researchers investigating the use of marijuana as an antiemetic with chemotherapy patients (Kutz et al., 1980; Morrow et al., 1982). Kutz and his colleagues found that patients initially reported that marijuana helped reduce postchemotherapy nausea/emesis; however, subsequent to repeated use of marijuana following chemotherapy treatments, patients began to notice that the odor of marijuana cigarettes in social settings made them slightly nauseated. For some patients, the taste or smell of marijuana became extremely aversive, eliciting nausea and emesis. Regardless of how it was presented (in a cookie, brownie, or cigarette), marijuana produced the aversive side effects it was intended to control. Morrow (1982) observed an even more dramatic example of inadvertent aversive conditioning. Some of his patients actually became nauseated in anticipation of consuming the THC tablet that had originally been prescribed to reduce chemotherapy side effects.

Based on the published data and clinical observations available, it appears to us most useful to view the nausea and emesis experienced by many patients in anticipation of chemotherapy infusions within the framework provided by the respondent conditioning paradigm. The development of anticipatory side effects seems to parallel laboratory demonstrations that noningestive environmental cues can assume aversive properties through association with illness (Best, Best, & Henggeler, 1977). This parallel is an imperfect one, however, since the presence of the aversion is inferred on different bases in the two situations. In the experimental situation, the extent of the aversion is determined by the extent to which the laboratory animal avoids the critical stimulus presumably associated with illness. In the chemotherapy situation, the patient is not routinely given the opportunity to avoid the stimuli associated with the chemotherapy treatment and which presumably becomes associated with later illness. As a result, patients are directly exposed to the aversive conditioned stimulus on a regular basis. Consequently, the presence of the conditioned aversion is not inferred on the basis of their tendency to avoid stimuli in the chemotherapy environment, but rather on the extent to which they exhibit nausea/emesis in response to the aversive conditioned stimulus. This reaction is identical to what Pavlov (1927) observed in dogs exposed to repeated injections of apomorphine.

PREDISPOSING FACTORS

Our knowledge of the factors that determine which patients will develop anticipatory nausea and vomiting is quite limited. At least 20 different variables have been studied in seven separate studies. The most fruitful lines of research have focused on the relationship between the development of aversion reactions to stimuli associated with chemotherapy and: (1) severity of nausea and vomiting following previous infusions; (2) number of chemotherapy sessions completed; (3) patient age; (4) presence of taste sensations and/or anxiety during previous infusions; and (5) patient coping style. Before reviewing this research it is important to point out that most of the research has been retrospective in nature and that assessments were generally made at a single point during the course of treatments. It is, therefore, quite possible that patients' experiences at the time of assessment might have influenced their recollections and that other relationships might have emerged if assessments had been completed at a later point in treatment. Given these limitations, it is reassuring to note that in general researchers have replicated one another's findings.

Severity of Posttreatment Side Effects

The most frequent finding has been a strong association between the severity, duration, and frequency of posttreatment nausea and vomiting and the development of pretreatment reactions (Cohen et al., 1982; Ingle, Burish, & Wallston, 1984; Morrow, 1982; Nesse et al., 1980; Nicholas, 1982; Rosencweig, Von Hoff, Slavik, & Muggia, 1977; Scogna & Smalley, 1979; Wilcox et al., 1980). Among patients receiving the same chemotherapy protocol, those who report either longer, more frequent, or more severe bouts of nausea and vomiting following each treatment are more likely to develop anticipatory reactions.

Two correlates follow from this relationship. First, patients receiving highly emetic drugs are at great risk for developing anticipatory reactions. For example, as was indicated in our discussion of prevalence, patients receiving cisplatin are at great risk, since cisplatin is the chemotherapy drug which currently produces the most severe posttreatment side effects. Second, patients entering on protocols which incorporate relatively large numbers of chemotherapeutic agents are at greater risk (Laszlo, 1983; Morrow, 1982), since such protocols are generally associated with more severe posttreatment side effects. Thus, it appears that the presence of any factor that increases the emeticity of a protocol increases the likelihood that patients will experience nonpharmacological side effects.

Number of Previous Chemotherapy Infusions

Another fairly general finding is that the patient's risk of developing anticipatory reactions increases as a function of the number of previous chemotherapy infusions (Nesse et al., 1980). This relationship has also appeared in the senior author's preliminary research with adolescents receiving chemotherapy before surgery for bone cancers. Medical chart reviews and patient interviews have been conducted with 90 patients. Initial analyses suggest that the probability of anticipatory side effects is approximately three times greater for children undergoing a second series of repeated chemotherapy infusions than for children undergoing their first course of treatment. Although this research has not been completed and more extensive analyses are scheduled, our findings are consistent with those obtained with adult patients.

Patient Age

It has generally been found that the younger the patient, the greater the risk of anticipatory reactions (Cohen et al., 1982; Ingle et al., 1984; Morrow, 1982). Unfortunately, we do not have a clear understanding of why this is the case. Research published to date has not contained sample sizes large enough to permit the statistical analyses necessary to identify the impact of variables associated with patient age. However, investigators working in the area have suggested four possible explanations. One is the fact that younger patients are more frequent victims of cancers (e.g., testicular) that are treated with highly emetic drugs (Laszlo, 1983). Thus, as a group, younger patients may experience greater posttreatment side effects and, perhaps because of that, are at greater risk for anticipatory reactions. Another possibility concerns the trend within clinical oncology to treat younger patients with more aggressive protocols. The rationale is that younger patients are generally stronger and are better able to withstand the physical side effects. Thus, younger patients may be at greater risk simply because they receive more emetic chemotherapeutic agents. The third and fourth explanations do not follow as closely from the existing body of research as the first two; they are clearly speculative in nature. It has been suggested, though not demonstrated, that younger patients may have different physiological reactions to the treatment than older individuals, and that these reactions are more likely to lead to nausea and vomiting. Also, younger patients may approach treatment with greater apprehension, distress, and anxiety, which in turn may also facilitate the development of nonpharmacological nausea/vomiting. Thus, it is possible that for younger patients chemotherapy represents a different physiological and emotional experience. Each of these hypotheses requires further examination, involving prospective analyses with large numbers of patients. Researchers generally agree that subsequent investigations must carefully isolate variables which change with age as most view age as an indirect risk factor.

Presence of Taste Sensations or Anxiety

An interesting series of findings concerns the relationship between sensations experienced during chemotherapy infusions and the development of anticipatory side effects. Prospective research by Love, Nerenz, and Leventhal (1982) revealed that patients who reported strong taste sensations as the chemotherapy drugs were being injected were more likely to manifest anticipatory nausea and vomiting later in the course of treatment. This relationship may result from a mediating effect of the taste sensation. That is, the taste sensations may facilitate the respondent conditioning by helping to bridge the interval between the conditioned stimulus and the unconditioned response (i.e., posttreatment nausea and vomiting). The taste sensation may also serve as a salient conditioned stimulus in its own right.

Anxiety during initial chemotherapy infusions has also been found in most studies to be associated with the development of anticipatory side effects (Altmaier, Ross, & Moore, 1982; Coons, 1982; Love, Nerenz, & Leventhal, 1982; Nerenz, Leventhal, Love, Coons, & Ringler, 1982), though there are some exceptions (e.g., Zook & Yasko, 1983). Patients who reported feeling anxious (i.e., upset, nervous, tense) during chemotherapy injections were more likely to develop anticipatory reactions. These results are consistent with those of Van Komen and Redd (1983) who found that patients who could be characterized (via state-trait anxiety scales) as being anxious were more likely to develop anticipatory side effects. Patients with relatively high trait anxiety scores were also more likely to experience chemotherapy infusions as distressful, unpleasant, and depressing than were patients with low trait anxiety scores.

The role of anxiety and the development of anticipatory reactions introduces a rather complex and unproven hypothesis: namely, Spence's (1958, 1964) notion of a positive association between conditionability and anxiety. Spence's conditionability-anxiety hypothesis is derived from Hullian learning theory (Hull, 1943) and Pavlovian notions concerning the physiological bases of personality (see Teplov, 1964). Specifically, trait anxiety scores are presumed to be positively related to an individual's generalized drive level. This is because drive level is presumed to be a function of the strength of the emotional response an individual experiences when confronted by noxious stimulation. The strength of this emotional response is presumably higher and more stable in patients with high trait anxiety, and hence their generalized drive level is higher. Generalized drive contributes to an increase in excitatory potential which, in turn, partially determines the strength of any response. According to Pavlov (see Teplov, 1964), increased excitatory potential, characteristic of the "weak" nervous system in humans, facilitates classical conditioning.

Although the evidence that trait anxiety is positively related to conditionability was described by Spence (1964) as "substantial," it must be kept in mind that there is considerable interindividual variation in performance on experimental conditioning tasks, and Spence (1964) himself acknowledged that the anxiety variable may only account for a small proportion of this variance.

Coping Style

An important and relatively unresearched factor in the development of chemotherapy side effects may be the patients' methods of coping with treatment. As Taylor (1982) found in her study of women faced with breast cancer, many patients discover effective means of controlling or reducing chemotherapy side effects on their own. In her research, Taylor noted that many of the chemotherapy patients interviewed reported using meditation, directed breathing, and self-relaxation to reduce nausea and vomiting. Indeed, in our clinical work we have met patients who listen to music, chew sweet candy, and/or "try to think of something else" to fight the nausea. Although we have not found patients who instituted such methods to prevent the symptoms from occurring in the first place, it is possible that there are patients who do so. It would be both clinically important and theoretically interesting if we could alter the risk of patients' developing anticipatory reactions by teaching them coping methods to be used *before* the symptoms appeared.

In summary, we suggest that an assessment of the emetic potential of the chemotherapy drugs, the resultant strength of the conditioning experience, and individual differences in coping style may allow a fairly accurate prediction of which patients will develop conditioned side effects. In this assessment, it is necessary to weigh each of the factors differently. That is, although each factor will be present to some degree in each patient, the factors will not be equal in their influence. As suggested previously, for example, a high emetic potential of the chemotherapy drugs may be sufficient for the development of conditioned responses regardless of the strength of the other factors. Future research is needed to determine the validity and importance of the factors hypothesized to predispose patients to develop nonpharmacologic side effects, and the nature of their interactions.

CONCLUSIONS

Many cancer patients display chemotherapy side effects that appear to be nonpharmacological in nature. That is, they experience severe nausea and/or vomiting before the drugs are infused. Of the several hypotheses that have been proposed to explain the etiology of nonpharmacological anticipatory side effects, the one that appears the most viable is that based on respondent conditioning. Through repeated association with postchemotherapy side effects, the sights, smells, tastes, and even thoughts associated with the treatment elicit nausea and vomiting. Although anticipatory side effects are clearly quite common, because of methodological problems in the research that has been conducted in the area it is impossible to state their actual prevalence. Well-designed research is needed to determine the prevalence rates for particular chemotherapy regimens, for particular types of cancers, and for particular types of patients. Moreover, these rates should be determined at regular intervals during the course of repeated treatments. At least five factors may be important in the development of anticipatory side effects. They include: (1) severity of nausea and vomiting following previous treatments; (2) number of chemotherapy sessions completed; (3) patient age; (4) presence of strong taste sensations and/or anxiety during initial chemotherapy infusions; and (5) patient coping style.

The repeated and systematic administration of highly toxic drugs to humans offers an excellent opportunity for clinically meaningful and theoretically important research. It also permits the examination of respondent conditioning theories of fears, taste aversions, and their treatment. Parameters of the phenomenon and the role of cognitive mediation can be systematically analyzed. Behavioral research on chemotherapy side effects thus represents a rich blend of scientific inquiry and humanitarian endeavor for the behavioral sciences.

ACKNOWLEDGMENT

The writing of this chapter was supported in part by a grant from the National Cancer Institute (CA 25516). The authors thank G. Andresen, M. Carey, R. Henderson, C. Hendler, and C. Neff for their helpful comments on an earlier draft of the manuscript.

REFERENCES

Altmaier, E. M., Ross, W. E., & Moore, K. (1982). A pilot investigation of the psychologic function of patients with anticipatory vomiting. *Cancer, 49*, 201–204.

Best, P. J., Best, M. R., & Henggeler, S. (1977). The contribution of environmental non-ingestive cues in conditioning with aversive internal consequence. In L. M. Barker, M. R. Best, and M. Domjan (Eds.), *Learning mechanisms in food selections.* Waco, TX: Baylor University Press.

Burish, T. G., & Carey, M. P. (1984). Conditioned responses to cancer chemotherapy: Etiology and treatment. In B. H. Fox & B. H. Newberry (Eds.), *Impact of psychoendocrine systems in cancer and immunity.* New York: C. J. Hogrefe.

Burish, T. G., & Lyles, J. N. (1979). Effectiveness of relaxation training in reducing the aversiveness of chemotherapy in the treatment of cancer. *Behavior Therapy and Experimental Psychiatry, 10*, 357–361.

Chang, J. C. (1981). Nausea and vomiting in cancer patients: An expression of psychological mechanisms? *Psychosomatics, 22*, 707–709.

Cohen, R. E., Sheehan, A., Ruckdeschel, J. C., & Blanchard, E. B. (1982). *The prediction of posttreatment and anticipatory nausea and vomiting associated with antineoplastic chemotherapy.* Paper presented at the Meeting of the Society of Behavioral Medicine, March, Chicago.

Collins, K. H., & Tatum, A. L. (1925). A conditioned salivary reflex established by chronic morphine poisoning. *American Journal of Physiology, 74*, 14–15.

Coons, H. L. (1982). *Conditioned nausea in cancer patients receiving Cisplatinum chemotherapy.* Unpublished manuscript. University of Wisconsin, Madison.

Fetting, J. H., Wilcox, P. M., Iwata, B. A., Criswell, E. L., Bosmajian, L. S., & Sheidler, V. R. (1983). Anticipatory nausea and vomiting in an ambulatory oncology population. *Cancer Treatment Reports, 67*, 1093–1098.

Fordyce, W. E. (1973). An operant conditioning method for managing chronic pain. *Post-Graduate Medicine, 53*, 123–124.

Garb, J. D., & Strunkard, A. J. (1974). Taste aversions in man. *American Journal of Psychiatry, 131*, 1204–1207.

Garcia, J., Kimeldorf, D. J., & Koelling, R. A. (1955). Conditioned aversion to saccharin resulting from exposure to gamma radiation. *Science, 122,* 157–158.

Garcia, J., McGowan, B. K., & Green, K. R. (1972). Biological constraints on conditioning. In M. E. P. Seligman & J. L. Hager (Eds.), *Biological boundaries of learning.* New York: Appleton-Century-Crofts.

Golden, S. (1975). Cancer chemotherapy and management of patient problems. *Nursing Forum, 12,* 279–303.

Hull, C. L. (1943). *Principles of behavior.* New York: Appleton-Century Crofts.

Ingersoll, B., & Curry, F. (1977). Rapid treatment of persistent vomiting in a 14-year-old female by shaping and time-out. *Journal of Behavior Therapy and Experimental Psychiatry, 8,* 305–307.

Katahn, M. (1967). Systematic desensitization and counseling for anxiety in a college basketball player. *Journal of Special Education, 1,* 309–313.

Katkin, E. S. (1976). Instrumental autonomic conditioning. In J. T. Spence, R. C. Carson, & J. W. Thibaut (Eds.), *Behavioral approaches to therapy.* Morristown, NJ: General Learning Press.

Katz, E. R. (1982). Behavioral conditioning in the development and maintenance of vomiting in cancer patients. *Psychosomatics, 23,* 650–651.

Katz, E. R., Kellerman, J. & Siegel, S. E. (1980). Behavioral distress in children with cancer undergoing medical procedures: Developmental considerations. *Journal of Consulting and Clinical Psychology, 48,* 356–365.

Ingle, R. J., Burish, T. G., & Wallston, K. A. (1984). Conditionability of cancer chemotherapy patients. *Oncology Nursing Forum, 11,* 97–102.

Kutz, I., Borysenko, J. Z., Come, S. E., & Benson, H. (1980). Paradoxical emetic response to antiemetic treatment in cancer patients. *New England Journal of Medicine, 303,* 1480.

Lacey, J. I. (1967). Somatic response patterning and stress: Some revisions of activation theory. In M. H. Appley & R. Trumball (Eds.), *Psychological stress.* New York: McGraw-Hill.

Laszlo, J. (1983). Emesis as limiting toxicity in cancer chemotherapy. In J. Laszlo (Ed.), *Antiemetics and cancer chemotherapy.* Baltimore: Williams and Wilkins.

Love, R. R., Nerenz, D. R., & Leventhal, H. (1982). The development of anticipatory nausea during cancer chemotherapy. *Proceedings of the American Society of Clinical Oncology,* April, St. Louis, MO.

Morrow, G. R. (1982). Prevalence and correlates of anticipatory nausea and vomiting in chemotherapy patients. *Journal of the National Cancer Institute, 68,* 484–488.

Morrow, G. R., Arseneau, J. C., Asbury, R. F., Bennett, J. M., & Boros, L. (1982). Anticipatory nausea and vomiting with chemotherapy. *New England Journal of Medicine, 306,* 431–432.

Nerenz, D. R., Leventhal, H., & Love, R. R. (1982). Factors contributing to emotional distress during cancer chemotherapy. *Cancer, 50,* 1020–1027.

Nerenz, D. R., Leventhal, H., Love, R. R., Coons, H., & Ringler, K. (1982). *Anxiety and taste of drugs during injections as predictors of anticipatory nausea in cancer chemotherapy.* Unpublished manuscript, University of Wisconsin, Madison.

Nesse, R. M., Carli, T., Curtis, G. C., & Kleinman, P. D. (1980). Pretreatment nausea in cancer chemotherapy: A conditioned response? *Psychosomatic Medicine, 42,* 33–36.

Nicholas, D. R. (1982). Prevalence of anticipatory nausea and emesis in cancer chemotherapy patients. *Journal of Behavioral Medicine, 5,* 461–463.

Pavlov, I. P. (1927). *Conditioned reflexes: An investigation of physiological activity of the cerebral cortex (Lecture III).* Oxford, England: Oxford University Press.

Penta, J., Poster, D., Bruno, S., & Jacobs, E. M. (1983). The pharmacologic treatment of nausea and vomiting caused by chemotherapy: A review. In J. Laszlo (Ed.), *Antiemetics and cancer chemotherapy.* Baltimore: Williams and Wilkins.

Redd, W. H., & Andresen, G. V. (1981). Conditioned aversion in cancer patients. *The Behavior Therapist, 4,* 3–4.

Riley, A. L., & Clarke, C. (1977). Conditioned taste aversions: A bibliography. In L. M. Barker, M. R. Best, & M. Domjam (Eds.), *Learning mechanisms in food selection.* Waco, TX: Baylor University Press.

Rosencweig, M., Von Hoff, D. D., Slavik, M., & Muggia, F. M. (1977). Cis-diammine dichloro platinum (II): A new anticancer drug. *Annals of Internal Medicine, 86,* 803–812.

Schulz, L. S. (1980). Classical (Pavlovian) conditioning of nausea and vomiting in cancer chemotherapy. *Proceedings of the American Society of Clinical Oncology, 21,* C–246.

Scogna, D. M., & Smalley, R. V. (1979). Chemotherapy induced nausea and vomiting. *American Journal of Nursing,* 1562–1564.

Seligman, M. E. P. (1970). On the generality of the laws of learning. *Psychological Review, 77,* 406–418.

Spence, K. W. (1958). A theory of emotionally based drive (D) and its relation to performance in simple learning situations. *American Psychologist, 13,* 131–141.

Spence, K. W. (1964). Anxiety (drive) level and performance in eyelid conditioning. *Psychological Bulletin, 61,* 129–139.

Swanson, D. W., Swenson, W. M., Huizenga, K. A., & Melson, S. J. (1976). Persistent nausea without organic cause. *Mayo Clinic Proceedings, 51,* 257–262.

Taylor, S. E. (1982). Social cognition and health. *Personality and Social Psychology Bulletin, 8,* 549–562.

Teplov, B. M. (1964). Problems in the study of general types of higher nervous activity in man and animals. In J. A. Gray (Ed.), *Pavlov's typology* (pp. 3–153). Oxford, England: Pergamon Press.

Van Komen, R. A., & Redd, W. H. (1983). Factors associated with anticipatory nausea/vomiting in women receiving cyclophosphamide, methotrexate, and 5-FU (CMF) adjuvant chemotherapy for breast carcinoma. *Cancer Treatment Reports, 66,* 1601–1604.

Wilcox, P. M., Fetting, J. H., Nettesheim, K. M., & Abeloff, M. D. (1982). Anticipatory vomiting in women receiving cyclophosphamide, methotrexate, and 5-FU (CMF) adjuvant chemotherapy for breast carcinoma. *Cancer Treatment Reports, 66,* 1601–1604.

Zook, D. J., & Yasko, J. M. (1983). Psychological factors: Their effect on nausea and vomiting experienced by clients receiving chemotherapy. *Oncology Nursing Forum, 10,* 76–81.

III IMPROVING THE NUTRITIONAL STATUS OF CANCER PATIENTS AND HIGH-RISK POPULATIONS

8 Nutritional Problems in Cancer Patients: Overview and Perspective

William DeWys, M.D.
Division of Cancer Prevention and Control, National Cancer Institute

INTRODUCTION

The major prognostic factors in cancer patients include tumor type, stage of disease, weight loss, and performance status (DeWys et al., 1980). Of these factors, weight loss is potentially the most amenable to therapeutic intervention and/or preventive intervention, and therefore is an important topic for further scientific inquiry. In this chapter I review data which delineates the prognostic effect of weight loss in cancer patients in terms of duration of survival and response to chemotherapy. I discuss the pathophysiology of weight loss in cancer patients and provide a background for understanding specific mechanisms of weight loss, such as learned food aversions and conditioned responses to therapy in cancer patients. The final portion of this chapter deals with nutritional intervention in support of the cancer patient.

INCIDENCE OF WEIGHT LOSS IN CANCER PATIENTS

In order to explore the extent of weight loss in cancerpatients we collected data on pretreatment weight loss from patients who were entering prospective clinical trials of cancer chemotherapy (DeWys, Begg, Lavin, Band, Bennett, Bertino, Cohen, Douglass, Engstrom, Horton, Johnson, Moertel, Oken, Perlia, Rosenbaum, Silverstein, Skell, Sponza, Tormey, 1980). At the time of study these patients had extensive disease judged to be beyond the scope of curative surgery or radiation therapy. Patients were interviewed to determine the percentage of body weight they had lost during the six months prior to the chemotherapy trial.

Some of these patients had had previous surgery or radiation therapy but they had not received chemotherapy. Therefore, the weight loss was not chemotherapy-related, but rather, was due to the disease effects of cancer as well as the effects of prior surgery or radiation therapy. As shown in Table 8.1, the frequency of weight loss ranged from 30% in patients with favorable non-Hodgkin's lymphoma to nearly 90% of patients with gastric cancer (DeWys et al., 1980). Note that the tumor types (pancreas and gastric) most frequently associated with weight loss also led to the greatest degree (>10%) of weight loss among the patients studied.

The differences in incidence and severity of weight loss from one tumor to another may reflect differences in the natural history of the different tumors. Patients with tumor types associated with a low incidence of weight loss may receive medical attention relatively early in the course of their disease before weight loss has occurred. For example, breast cancer, lymphoma, and sarcoma are often located near the body surface so that the presence of the primary tumor leads to early self-detection. In contrast, cancer arising in the pancreas and the stomach is deep inside the body and is not amenable to early detection.

TABLE 8.1
Frequency of Weight Loss in Cancer Patients

Tumor Type	Patients (no.)	Weight Loss in the Previous 6 mos. (%)[a] 0	0-5	5-10	>10
Favorable non-Hodgkin's lymphoma[b]	290	69	14	8	10
Breast	289	64	22	8	6
Acute nonlymphocytic leukemia	129	61	27	8	4
Sarcoma	189	60	21	11	7
Unfavorable non-Hodgkin's lymphoma[c]	311	52	20	13	15
Colon	307	46	26	14	14
Prostate	78	44	28	18	10
Lung, small cell	436	43	23	20	14
Lung, nonsmall cell	590	39	25	21	15
Pancreas[d]	111	17	29	28	26
Nonmeasurable gastric	179	17	21	32	30
Measurable gastric	138	13	20	29	38
Total	3,047	46	22	17	15

[a] Data shown are percentage of line total in each weight loss category.
[b] The favorable non-Hodgkin's lymphoma protocal includes nodular lymphocytic well differentiated, nodular lymphocytic poorly differentiated, nodular mixed, nodular histiocytic, and diffuse lymphocytic well differentiated.
[c] The unfavorable non-Hodgkin's lymphoma protocal includes diffuse lymphocytic poorly differentiated, diffuse mixed, diffuse histiocytic, diffuse undifferentiated, and mycosis fungoides.
[d] Data for pancreatic cancer are weight loss in previous 2 mos.

TABLE 8.2
Effect of Weight Loss on Survival

Tumor Type	Median Survival (weeks)		
	No Weight Loss	Weight Loss[a]	P Value[b]
Favorable non-Hodgkin's lymphoma	*c*	138	<0.01
Breast	70	45	<0.01
Acute nonlymphocytic leukemia	8	4	N.S.
Sarcoma	46	25	<0.01
Unfavorable non-Hodgkin's lymphoma	107	55	<0.01
Colon	43	21	<0.01
Prostate	46	24	<0.05
Lung, small cell	34	27	<0.05
Lung, nonsmall cell	20	14	<0.01
Pancreas	14	12	N.S.
Nonmeasurable gastric	41	27	<0.05
Measurable gastric	18	16	N.S.

[a]All categories of weight loss (0-5% and 10%) have been combined.
[b]The P values refer to a test of the hypothesis that the entire survival curves are identical, not merely a test of the medians. However, in all disease sites under study, the median is a representative indicator of the survival distribution, and consequently its use as a summary statistic is acceptable.
[c]Only 20 of 199 patients have died, so median survival cannot be estimated. However, the observed rate of failure predicts that the survival will be significantly longer than for the group with weight loss.

PROGNOSTIC EFFECT OF WEIGHT LOSS

To evaluate the prognostic effect of prechemotherapy weight loss, we compared the survival of patients who had lost weight to that of patients with the same type of cancer who had not lost weight. As shown in Table 8.2, for each tumor type evaluated, survival was shorter in patients who had experienced weight loss than in patients who had not (DeWys et al., 1980). In nine of 12 comparisons this difference was statistically significant. For several tumors (sarcoma, unfavorable non-Hodgkin's lymphoma, colon cancer and prostate cancer) the median survival was approximately twice as long in patients who had not lost weight as in the patients who had. When the data were analyzed by degree of weight loss, a greater shortening of survival was associated with greater degrees of weight loss (Table 8.3) (DeWys et al., 1980). For many tumors, the greatest difference was between the no weight loss group and the 0–5% weight loss category, as shown for prostate cancer and colorectal cancer in Table 8.3.

TABLE 8.3
Effect of Weight Loss Subcategories on Median Survival

Tumor Type	Median Survival (wk)				
		Weight Loss			
	None	0-5%	5-10%	>10%	*P* Value
Nonsmall cell lung	20	17	13	11	<0.01
Prostate	46	30	18	9	<0.05
Colorectal	43	27	15	20	<0.01

[a] Based on a simultaneous statistical test of the null hypothesis that median survival is not affected by weight loss.

We wondered whether the impact of weight loss was simply an impact of greater tumor extent. In other words, were the patients who had lost weight simply patients with more advanced disease, and could this explain their shorter survival? Representative data relative to this question are shown in Table 8.4 for patients with colon cancer. Tumor involvement was coded as absent or present for three anatomic sites (liver, lung, and bone), and this number was taken as an approximation of total tumor volume. As shown in Table 8.4, for each tumor volume category, survival was shorter for patients with weight loss compared to those without weight loss. A similar pattern was observed in breast, prostate, and nonmeasurable gastric cancer. In addition, in three tumor categories (non-small cell lung cancer, small cell lung cancer, and sarcoma) weight loss had a prognostic effect in patients with limited tumor extent, but in patients with more advanced tumor extent, weight loss did not affect survival (DeWys et al., 1980).

Because weight loss was found to affect survival we wondered whether it would also affect the pattern of response to chemotherapy. Pretreatment weight loss was associated with a lower frequency of response to chemotherapy (complete remission plus partial remission) in four tumor categories (breast cancer, acute leukemia, colon cancer, non-small cell lung cancer). However only in breast cancer did this difference reach statistical significance (DeWys et al., 1980; DeWys, Begg, Band & Tormey, 1982). As shown in Table 8.5, the overall response rate for patients with breast cancer who had not lost weight was 61%, that for patients with weight loss was 43%. A difference was also seen in the complete response rate (CR) with 18% complete remission in patients without weight loss compared with only 7% in patients who had had previous weight loss (DeWys et al., 1982).

An analysis of the interaction of disease extent, weight loss, and response to chemotherapy in breast cancer showed a consistently lower response rate for patients with weight loss compared to those without weight loss within each tumor extent category (Table 8.6). The impact of weight loss on response was approximately equal to the impact of tumor extent (compare no visceral metastases, weight loss group vs. $\geq$ 2 visceral metastases, no weight loss group). Weight loss also affected the likelihood of a complete response to chemotherapy within each tumor extent category (Table 8.7) (DeWys et al., 1982).

TABLE 8.4
Effect on Median Survival of Weight Loss and Tumor Extent for Colon Cancer

	No Weight Loss		Weight Loss		
Tumor Extent	Median Survival (wk)	Patients (no.)	Median Survival (wk)	Patients (no.)	P Value for Survival Difference
0	52	60	31	51	0.05
1	37	75	19	101	0.01
2	25	6	14	14	NS

TABLE 8.5
Effect of Weight Loss on Response to Chemotherapy for Breast Cancer

Weight Loss	No. of Patients With Response/No. treated		
	CR	PR	CR+PR
No	37/210(18%)	91/210(43%)	128/210(61%)
Yes	8/120(7%)	44/120(37%)	52/120(43%)
(*p* value)	(*p*=0.01)	NS[a]	(*p*=0.01)

[a]Not significant

TABLE 8.6
Effect of Disease Extent and Weight Loss on Overall Response to Chemotherapy in Breast Cancer [a]

	No. of Responses (CR+PR) No. of Patients Treated	
Viceral Metastases	No Weight Loss	Weight Loss
0	40/61 (66%)	12/22 (55%)
1	59/97 (61%)	24/51 (47%)
≥2	29/52 (56%)	16/47 (34%)

[a]*p*=0.01

TABLE 8.7
Effect of Disease Extent and Weight Loss on CR to Chemotherapy in Breast Cancer [a]

	No. of CR No. of Patients Treated	
Viceral Metastases	No Weight Loss	Weight Loss
0	14/61 (23%)	4/22 (18%)
1	16/97 (16%)	2/51 (4%)
≥2	7/52 (13%)	2/47 (4%)

[a]*p*=0.01

PATHOPHYSIOLOGY OF WEIGHT LOSS IN CANCER PATIENTS

The pathophysiology of weight loss in cancer patients is not entirely understood but can be explained in part by consideration of energy balance, altered carbohydrate metabolism, and altered protein metabolism (DeWys, 1982). Energy balance in the cancer patient may be negative because of decreased caloric intake, increased caloric expenditure or a combination of these two factors. DeWys, Costa, and Henkin (1981) used 3-day diet diaries to measure caloric intake in cancer patients. Patients recorded the foods they ate and the amount of each consumed using standard household measures. From these diaries, calories were calculated using a computer program and USDA data on food composition (DeWys et al., 1981). As a reference for assessment of the adequacy of caloric intake the basal energy requirement was calculated using the Harris-Benedict equation. This equation takes into account the effect of height, weight, age, and sex on basal energy expenditure. A moderate level of activity requires a caloric intake about 50% above the basal energy requirements (150% of basal energy requirements). Only 30% of patients had a caloric intake which was sufficient to meet the needs for basal energy expenditure plus a moderate level of activity (Figure 8.1). In 40% of patients, the energy intake was greater than calculated for basal energy expenditure, but less than that required for a moderate level of activity. In 25% of patients, the caloric intake was below the calculated basal energy expenditure (DeWys et al., 1981).

Symptoms that might interfere with eating were assessed through questionnaire interviews given to a series of 169 cancer patients (DeWys et al., 1981).

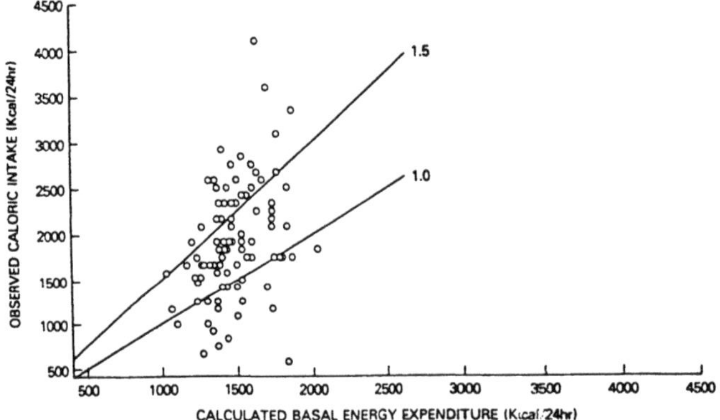

FIG. 8.1. Correlation between observed caloric intake and calculated basal energy expenditure. The line labeled 1.0 is the line of identity of caloric intake and basal energy expenditure and the line 1.5 represents caloric intake 50% above basal expenditure.

TABLE 8.8
Symptoms That Might Interfere With Eating

Symptom	No. of Patients Reporting this Symptom
Altered small	21
Smell loss	10
Altered taste	53
Taste loss	17
Chewing problem	13
Soreness in mouth	7
Dryness in mouth	14
Swallowing problem	15
Nausea	9
Vomiting	4
GI obstruction	5
Fill up quickly	22
Constipation	6
Diarrhea	4
Pain	14
Infection	1
Don't feel like eating	29
Side effects of chemotherapy	15
Side effects of radiation	3
Psychosocial	7
Socioeconomic	1
Metabolic	6
Others	8

Alterations in taste and smell were the most frequently reported symptoms (see Table 8.8). Also of note were symptoms related to the gastrointestinal system, and of these, the most common was a report of a sense of filling up quickly, which might be expected to interfere with the size of a meal.

Multiple factors may be involved in decreased eating in cancer patients including metabolic factors discussed below. In addition, abnormalities of taste and smell sensation have been reported in cancer patients (DeWys and Walters, 1975 and DeWys, 1978). A frequent abnormality is an elevated threshold for sweet taste, observed in approximately one-fourth of patients studied. Other abnormalities include an increased sensitivity to bitter taste and an elevated threshold for salty taste (DeWys and Walters, 1975 and DeWys, 1978). The frequency of taste abnormalities increases with increasing tumor extent, but does not correlate with tumor cell type. The abnormalities are reversible with regression of the tumor, and they correlate with reduced caloric intake (DeWys, 1978). Learned aversions related to taste may contribute to decreased eating of specific foods (Bernstein & Webster, this volume; Smith, Blumsack, & Bilek, this volume). The extent to which these learned aversions contribute to a decrease in caloric intake in cancer patients is not clear.

Energy expenditure in cancer patients has been studied with a variety of techniques including indirect and direct calorimetry. Indirect calorimetry involves measuring oxygen consumption and carbon dioxide production and deriving energy expenditure from appropriate mathematical formulas. In direct calorimetry, energy expenditure is measured by directly measuring body heat production. These studies can be summarized as showing modest increases in caloric expenditure in cancer patients with observed values being in the range of 20–50% higher than would be expected based on the subject's age, sex, body size, and activity level (DeWys & Kisner, 1982; Knox, Crosby, Feurer, Buzby, Miller, & Mullen, 1983; Warnold, Lundholm, & Schersten, 1978).

The increased energy expenditure in cancer patients may have several explanations (DeWys, 1982). Cancer cells, like all living cells, utilize energy to transport nutrients and minerals from outside into the cells just to stay alive. In addition, cancer cells are growing and dividing to form new cancer cells, and this requires energy, especially for synthesis of cellular proteins. The nutrients which the tumor cells require for maintenance and for growth must go through the processes of ingestion, digestion, absorption, and circulation prior to reaching them and these processes require energy. As a tumor grows it stimulates the growth of normal host tissues, such as blood vessels and fibrous tissue, and this growth of normal tissues also requires extra energy. Finally, the tumor cells use the Cori cycle to derive energy from glucose and this cycle returns lactate to the circulation. This lactate is converted to glucose in the liver and kidney using an energy-requiring metabolic sequence (Holroyde & Reichard, 1981).

In a normal subject the Cori cycle is involved in the delivery of glucose to organs (muscle and red blood cells) which metabolize glucose only partially and return lactate to the circulation. The lactate is carried by the circulation to the liver and kidney where it is converted to glucose to complete the cycle. The conversion of lactate back to glucose in the liver and kidney is an energy-requiring process. In a normal person, this cycle supplies energy to muscle and red blood cells delivering approximately 70 grams of glucose per day. In the cancer bearing patient, the Cori cycle also delivers glucose into the tumor (several hundred grams per day) with a consequent increased delivery of lactate back to the liver and kidney. Increased Cori cycling correlates with the presence of weight loss in cancer patients (Holroyde & Reichard, 1981).

The role of the Cori cycle activity in learned food aversions in cancer patients should be studied. A learned aversion to a food could develop if ingestion of a food were followed by an unpleasant sensation. In cancer patients, when carbohydrate intake is increased, production of lactate increases to six or eight times the normal value, accompanied by an increase in plasma lactate (Holroyde, C. P., Myers, R. N., Smink, R. D., Putnam, R. C., Paul, P., & Reichard G. A., 1977). It is known from studies in normal volunteers that infusion of lactate produces a symptom complex that includes anorexia, nausea, and anxiety. Thus, one could envision that carbohydrate intake by a cancer patient would result in increased blood lactate levels, which would lead to the unpleasant symptoms of anorexia, nausea, and anxiety, which would serve as the stimulus for a conditioned aversion to intake of carbohydrate-rich foods.

Another alteration of metabolism in the cancer patient is decreased glucose tolerance, that is, an exaggerated response of the blood sugar to ingestion of a standard amount of glucose (DeWys and Kisner, 1982). If a normal person drinks a beverage containing a moderate amount of sugar (generally 75gm of glucose) the blood sugar rises briefly, followed by return to baseline levels within three hours of the intake of the glucose. Insulin production in a normal person also rises abruptly and then gradually tapers off. In contrast, in cancer patients, the rise in blood sugar continues for a longer period of time and takes a longer time to return to the baseline level; the output of insulin is somewhat delayed and reduced. The pathophysiology of the abnormalities in glucose tolerance in the cancer patient includes decreased insulin ouput and insulin resistance. The mechanism of the decreased insulin output, or of insulin resistance, is not well understood.

There are several implications of the altered glucose tolerance in cancer patients. One is the impact of altered blood glucose levels on appetite. Blood glucose is one of the factors that influence the appetite center and an elevated blood glucose may depress appetite. Because cancer patients may have abnormally long-lasting elevations in blood glucose following the ingestion of glucose-rich substances, they may show a correspondingly prolonged suppression of appetite after intake of carbohydrate. Further, blood glucose levels may be elevated for longer periods after a large meal than after the single intake of glucose in the glucose tolerance test. This pattern of elevation of blood glucose may provide a partial explanation for reduced appetite for meals, other than breakfast, often reported by cancer patients. The patient may be able to eat breakfast because his blood sugar has returned to normal overnight, but he lacks appetite later in the day due to the prolonged elevation of blood glucose following breakfast.

A second implication of the altered glucose tolerance in cancer patients is its potential impact on gastrointestinal function. An elevated blood glucose level may delay stomach emptying. Thus, in the cancer patient a prolonged elevation of blood glucose after a meal could provide a sense of fullness, resulting in further suppression of appetite. In this regard it is noteworthy that cancer patients frequently report a sensation of filling up quickly (Table 8.8).

PATHOPHYSIOLOGY OF MUSCLE WEAKNESS IN CANCER PATIENTS

As discussed in the introduction, activity level, or performance status, is an important prognostic factor in cancer patients. A decreased activity level in a cancer patient can be related most often to muscle weakness and muscle wasting.

As a background for understanding muscle weakness and muscle wasting, we need to review the biochemistry of protein metabolism in the cancer patient.

In a healthy person, the normal processes of cell renewal result in breakdown of old proteins and the synthesis of new proteins. The old proteins are broken down into amino acids, some of which are released into the circulation. New proteins are synthesized from amino acids, in part drawn from the breakdown of old proteins, and, in part derived from dietary sources.

In the cancer patient there is an increased breakdown of proteins in muscle, with a corresponding increase in release of amino acids into the circulation (Norton, Burt, & Brennan, 1980). In addition, there is an overall decrease in synthesis of protein within the muscle of cancer patients. Other alterations in protein synthesis are beyond the scope of this paper (Lundholm et al., 1979 and Lundholm, Ekman, Karlberg, Edstrom, & Shersten, 1980). Synthesis of protein in muscle tissue can be measured by following the incorporation of labeled amino acid into protein. Lundholm and his colleagues studied synthesis of muscle protein by taking muscle biopsy specimens from cancer patients and controls and measuring the incorporation of amino acids into the protein. They observed reduced protein synthesis in the muscle tissue from cancer patients (Lundholm, Bylund, Holm & Schersten, 1976). Based on the evidence for decreased insulin production in the cancer patient, they speculated that perhaps this depressed protein synthesis would be corrected by adding insulin. Consequently, they studied protein synthesis in muscle in the presence of increased insulin. Although added insulin did increase protein synthesis, the increase occurred in both the cancer patients and the controls with persistent differences between the cancer patients and the controls (Lundholm, Holm, Schersten, 1978). They concluded that the decreased protein synthesis in the cancer patient was not simply attributable to insufficient insulin. They also studied the effect of supplemental amino acids. Adding excess amino acids to muscle tissue *in vitro* increased protein synthesis in both the cancer patients and in the controls (Lundholm, et al., 1976). However, again the difference between normal subjects and cancer patient persisted. Therefore, the decreased protein synthesis in muscle in cancer patients appears not to be caused by either insufficient insulin or insufficient amino acids.

We turn now to a consideration of the muscle weakness and wasting of muscle in the cancer patient. Muscle wasting in cancer patients may be influenced by several factors. Tumor cells derive their energy requirements from anaerobic metabolism via the Cori cycle. The tumor cells use glucose rather than lipids as their main energy source. Many tissues in the body can metabolize fatty acids and glycerol through the Krebs cycle, but this cycle is deficient in tumor cells. A major source of glucose is food that is ingested. If the amount of glucose ingested is insufficient, (recall the decreased caloric intake in cancer patients, (Fig. 8.1) glycogen is broken down to supply glucose to the tumor. However, the body has a limited store of glycogen, and when that is exhausted, glucose is derived from metabolic conversion of amino acids. Because the largest reservoir of amino acids in the body is the skeletal muscle, they will be drawn from muscle to supply the glucose needs of the tumor. In addition, amino acids are drawn from the muscle to provide precursors for protein synthesis within the tumor. Thus, there are several mechanisms for loss of amino acids from muscle in cancer patients with resulting muscle weakness and wasting.

When a normal person loses weight by caloric restriction, generally more than three-quarters of the weight is lost from body fat and only a small amount from body muscle. In cancer patients, the weight loss comes almost equally from muscle and fat (Cohn, Gartenhaus, Sawitsky, Rai, Ellis, Yasumura, & Vartsky, 1981). Thus, there is much more wasting of muscle in a cancer patient than in a normal person.

NUTRITIONAL INTERVENTION IN CANCER PATIENTS

A number of questions need to be asked about nutritional support of cancer patients: Who should be treated? When should treatment be given? How much of the nutrient intake goes to the patient and how much to the tumor? One measure of the amount of nutrients being used by the tumor is the amount of lactate it produces. Holroyde et al. (1977) have documented increased lactate production in the tumor-bearing patients receiving parenteral nutrition. This increased lactate production suggests increased metabolic activity within the tumor in response to increased nutrient intake.

The overall goal of nutritional support of the cancer patient should be improvement of the patient's health which might increase the likelihood of a favorable response to therapy and aid the recovery from its adverse effects. Thus, the ultimate question becomes, does the nutritional supportive therapy result in improvement in survival of the cancer patient or stimulate tumor growth? Addressing the question of who should be treated, there is a continuum ranging from good candidates for nutritional supportive therapy, in whom decreased caloric intake is the major factor in weight loss, to poor candidates, in whom increased energy expenditure is the major factor. Decreased caloric intake can be remedied by nutritional supportive therapy, such as enteral or parenteral feeding. Although the energy required to satisfy increased expenditure could be provided, the increased food intake may further increase energy expenditure; a positive balance may prove elusive.

Regarding the question of when nutritional therapy should be given, one should consider the natural history of the disease and its responsiveness to therapy. In the ideal situation effective anticancer intervention (radiation, chemotherapy, etc.) is available so that the increased nutrition will benefit the host rather than simply supplying increased nutrients to the tumor. At the other end of the spectrum, patients for whom there is no effective anticancer treatment probably should not be considered for nutritional supportive therapy. The nutritional support may accelerate tumor metabolism, to the detriment of the host.

Finally, we consider whether nutritional supportive therapy results in improvement in patient response to therapy and/or improvement in survival. A number of studies have evaluated the role of parenteral nutrition as an adjunct to surgery in cancer patients. Although several small studies failed to show an advantage, a large, randomized, controlled clinical trial has shown that cancer patients had fewer surgical complications and decreased mortality when given parenteral nutrition before and after surgery compared to controls receiving similar surgery without preoperative parental nutrition (Mueller, Brenne, & Dienst, 1982).

In this study, patients with cancers arising in the gastrointestinal tract were randomly assigned to receive 10 days of preoperative parenteral nutrition (1.5gm amino acids/kg body weight and 11gm glucose/kg body weight per day) by a central venous catheter, or to receive a regular hospital diet. There were 66 patients in the parenteral nutrition group and 59 in the regular diet group. The incidence of major complications (intra-abdominal abscess, peritonitis, anastomatic leakage and ileus) was lower in the parenteral nutrition group (11/66) than in the regular diet group (19/59, $p < 0.05$). Also the mortality rate was lower for the parenteral nutrition group (3/66) compared to the regular diet group (11/59, $p < 0.05$). Postoperative pneumonia was more common in the regular diet group (23/59 vs. 20/66) and the course of the pneumonia was more severe in the regular diet group in which 12 required artificial respiration, compared with four in the parenteral nutrition group ($p < 0.05$). The mean weight gain between admission and surgery was 1.98 kg in the parenteral nutrition group; the controls lost 1.04 kg.

The results of this study suggest that preoperative parenteral nutrition may result in more rapid wound healing leading to a lower incidence of complications. In addition, preoperative parenteral nutrition may increase muscle strength which could explain the lower incidence of pneumonia and the lower frequency of use of artificial respiration in the parenteral nutrition group. Increased muscle strength may assist in coughing to clear pulmonary secretions thus preventing pneumonia, or decreasing its severity. In a setting in which the tumor can be removed, it appears that nutritional support results in improvement of the health of cancer patients. In studies of cancer patients receiving radiation therapy nutritional support has been shown to decrease or prevent weight loss, (Bothe, Valerio, Bistrian, & Blackburn, 1979), but no study has shown either improved response to therapy or improved survival. In patients receiving chemotherapy, adjunctive nutritional therapy may prevent weight loss and may reduce treatment delays related to more rapid recovery from toxicity (Clamon, DeWys, Kubota, Lininger, Kramer, Feld, Weiner, Moran, Blum, Evans, Jeejeebhoy & Giffen, 1982), but no large randomized controlled trial has shown either improved response rate or improved survival.

FUTURE DIRECTIONS

Although poor nutritional status correlates with a poor prognosis in cancer patients, efforts to improve nutritional status have had limited impact on prognosis in these patients. More research is needed in this area. Aspects which should be considered in a chemotherapy-related trial include the following:

1. Nutritional supplementation should be given over a sufficient duration of time, perhaps over several months. Many trials have used only a short duration of nutritional support (3–4 weeks), and weight gained during the period of supplementation is often rapidly lost thereafter.
2. The trials should include an exercise program. Increased caloric intake without exercise will result in deposition of fat, while calories plus exercise may rebuild depleted body muscle.
3. There should be emphasis on the schedule and intensity of chemotherapy given in conjunction with the nutritional support. If recovery from the toxicity from chemotherapy is hastened by nutritional support it may be possible to shorten the intervals between cycles of chemotherapy and thus increase the intensity of the chemotherapy.

REFERENCES

Bothe, A., Valerio, D., Bistrian, B. R., Blackburn, G. L. (1979). Randomized control trial of hospital nutritional support during abdominal radiotherapy. *Journal of Enteral Parenteral Nutrition, 3*, 292.

Clamon, G., DeWys, W., Kubota, T., Lininger, L., Kramer, B., Feld, R., Weiner, R., Moran, E., Blum, R., Evans, W. K., Jeejeebhoy, K., & Giffen, C. (1982). Hyeralimentation (IVH) as an adjunct to therapy for small cell lung cancer (SCCL): Preliminary report on safety and nutritional efficacy. *Proceedings of the American Society of Clinical Oncology.*

Cohn, S. H., Gartenhaus, W., Sawitsky, A., Rai, K., Ellis, K. J., Yasumura, S., & Vartsky, D. (1981). Compartmental body composition of cancer patients by measurement of total body nitrogen, potassium, and water. *Metab Clin Exp*, 1981, *30*, 222–229.

DeWys, W. D. (1978). Taste abnormalities and caloric intake in cancer patients: A review. *Journal of Human Nutrition, 32*, 447–453.

DeWys, W. D. (1982). Pathophysiology of cancer cachexia: Current understanding and areas for future research. *Cancer Research, 42*, 721s–726s.

DeWys, W. D., Begg, C. B., Band, P. R., & Torney, D. C. (1982). The impact of malnutrition on treatment results in breast cancer. *Cancer Treatment Report, 65*, 87–92.

DeWys, W. D., Begg, C., Lavin, P. T., et al. (1980). Prognostic effect of weight loss prior to chemotherapy in cancer patients. *American Journal of Medicine, 69*, 491–497.

DeWys, W. D., Costa, G., & Henkin, R. (1981). Clinical parameters related to anorexia. *Cancer Treatment Report, 65*, 49–52.

DeWys, W. D., & Kisner, D. (1982). Principles of nutritional care of cancer patient. In S. K. Carter, Glatstein, & R. B. Livingstone (Eds.), *Principles of cancer treatment* (pp. 252–259). New York: McGraw Hill.

DeWys, W. D., & Walters, K. (1975). Abnormalities of taste sensation in cancer patients. *Cancer 36*, 1888–1896.

Holroyde, C. P., Myers, R. N., Smink, R. D., Putnam, R. C., Paul, R., & Reichard, G. A. (1977). Metabolic response to total parenteral nutrition in cancer patients. *Cancer Research, 37,* 3109–3114.

Holroyde, C. P., & Reichard, G. A. (1981). Carbohydrate metabolism in cancer cachexia. *Cancer Treatment Report. 65*(5), 55–59.

Knox, L. A., Crosby, L. O., Feurer, I. D., Buzby, G. P., Miller, C. L., & Mullen, C. L. (1983). Energy expenditure in malnourished cancer patients. *Ann Surgery, 197,* 152–162.

Lundholm, K., Bylund, A. C., Holm, J., & Schersten, T. (1976). Skeletal muscle metabolism in patients with malignant tumor. *European Journal of Cancer, 12,* 465.

Lundholm, K., Ekman, L., Edstrom, S., Karlberg, I., Jagenburg, R., & Schersten, T. (1979). Protein synthesis in liver tissue under the influence of a methylcholanthrene induced sarcoma in mice. *Cancer Research, 39,* 4657–4661.

Lundholm, K., Ekman, L., Karlberg, I., Edstrom, S., & Schersten, T. (1980). Comparison of hepatic cathepsin D activity in response to tumor growth and to caloric restriction in mice. *Cancer Research, 40,* 1680–1685.

Mueller, J. M., Brenne, U., & Dienst, J. (1982). Preoperative parenteral feeding in patients with gastrointestinal cancer. *Lancet, I,* 68–71.

Norton, J. A., Burt, M. E., & Brennan, M. F. (1980). In vivo utilization of substrate by human sarcoma-bearing limbs. *Cancer, 45,* 2934–2939.

Warnold, I., Lundholm, K., & Schersten, T. (1978). Energy balance and body composition in cancer patients. *Cancer Research, 38,* 1801–1807.

9 Dietary Intervention in Cancer Prevention Trials and Clinical Practice: Some Methodological Issues

Elizabeth Bright-See, Ph.D.
Ludwig Institute for Cancer Research, Toronto Branch for Human Cancer Prevention

Sandra M. Levy, Ph.D.
School of Medicine, University of Pittsburgh

There are two issues of primary importance concerning diet and cancer: The possible role of dietary factors in the etiology of specific types of cancer, and diet as a component in the management and/or treatment of cancer patients. Related to the first issue, the variation in incidence and mortality from specific types of cancers between countries (Segi, 1980) and sometimes within countries (Ackerman, Weinstein, & Kaplan, 1978) suggests that many cancers are associated with dietary factors (Doll & Peto, 1981). Numerous epidemiological and animal studies have demonstrated associations between specific foods or food components and the risk of particular cancer (National Research Council, 1982).

Related to the second issue, weight loss in cancer patients is associated with poorer prognosis for long term survival (Chlebowski, Heber, & Block, 1983). The nutritional abnormalities associated with weight loss can have a direct effect on host status and tumor burden by, for example, altering hormonal and immunological factors. Nutritional deficit and cachexia can also indirectly affect the course of neoplasia by rendering the host unable to withstand the rigors of aggressive treatment.

The possible role of any dietary factor (whether nutrient, nonnutrient, additive, contaminant, or artifact of processing) in the prevention or treatment of human cancer is best tested using a methodological procedure called the randomized intervention trial. In this procedure, subjects are randomly assigned to either a group that receives a specific dietary intervention or to a group that does not (i.e., to a control group of some type). However, dietary trials face two basic methodological problems: How to assess eating behavior and how to design tools and strategies to change that behavior in a clearly defined manner. This discussion focuses on these methodological issues. Although the emphasis is on healthy and early-stage cancer subgroups, it should be noted that valid assessment of past and current diet in more advanced patients is no less difficult to obtain. And certainly factors such as compliance with nutritional health care plans are of major importance in studies of advanced cancer patients. In addition, side effects such as nausea could become conditioned to inpatient surroundings and nutritional deficits could be enhanced by such learned phenomena. Nevertheless, the focus of our discussion is healthy populations at risk for cancer development, with some additional comments concerning nutritional interventions in patient subgroups.

DIETARY ASSESSMENT: THE MEASUREMENT OF EATING BEHAVIOR

Common Methods: A Question of Purpose

There are several standard techniques for the measurement of diet in human populations (Krantzler, Mullen, Comstock, Holden, Schulz, Brevetti, & Meiselman 1982), and these various methods have recently been reviewed (Graham, 1980; Marshall, Priore, Haughey, Rzepka, & Graham, 1980; Murphy & Michael, 1982; Stunkard & Waxman, 1981). Block (1982) described the four most common methods of dietary assessment carried out in large population studies—diet history, 24-hour recall, 7-day recall, and 7-day record—and reviewed the reliability and validity studies associated with each method. The diet history, aimed at assessing the long term pattern of usual food intake, requires an extensive interview by a trained nutritionist. In this interview the nutritionist attempts to determine the frequency and amount of food category consumption over a lifetime or an extended segment of one's life. In the 24-hour recall method, the subject is asked to recall all food consumed over the last 24 hours; this method requires less time and less nutritional training for the interviewer. The 7-day recall is an attempt to capitalize on recent memory and tap a more representative sample of the subject's current eating behavior than merely the past 24-hours. The 7-day record requires a recording on the part of the subject of actual food intake, for a one-week period, estimating portion sizes or caloric consumption.

Block concluded that all of these methods have some degree of validity when measured against one another, as well as when measured against clinical criteria such as weight change. She also concluded that further attempts to perfect and validate these methods are desirable. "In doing so, it is important to gather as much information as possible on weight change and *changes in eating behavior*, so as to evaluate agreement or lack of it between independent, objective measures" (Block, 1982, p. 503, emphasis added).

Although Block favored continued research in this area, she also concluded that the current methods are good enough for large population studies of the association between diet and disease risk. However, if we move beyond large population, descriptive or analytical studies of association, to clinical intervention with patient or at-risk populations, then we could be concerned with a more precise measure of dietary behavior than has heretofore been required. That is, if we are concerned with the question of understanding disease mechanisms, we are going to have to measure as validly and precisely as possible what was eaten last year and last month, as well as yesterday, in order to target diet constituents to be modified and establish causal relationships that affect cancer risk status.

Stunkard and Waxman (1982) also reviewed the evidence on accuracy of self-report of food intake. They concluded that while many studies have been carried out on small and unrepresentative samples—and while such factors as age (Madden, Goodman, & Guture, 1976) and base weight (Spitzer & Rodin, 1981) seem to introduce response bias—the data suggest that self-reported 24-hour recall is fairly accurate. In their own study, they reported a strong linear relationship (r = .96) between measured food intake and the 24-hour dietary recall of food intake by obese and nonobese subjects. However, the subjects tended to over-report food intake when it was low, and under-report food intake when it was high. Although they found no difference in reporting as a function of base weight, others (Brownell, 1982; Goodstein, 1983) have found this individual difference factor to be of major importance in this regard.

Block (1982) stressed the importance of validating self-report against actual eating behavior. Schucker (1982) reported results from a pilot study assessing the validity of collecting diet history data via telephone rather than through personal interviews. In this study with college students, the validity of 6-hour and 24-hour telephone recalls of three to seven days of food consumption was compared to the validity of written records periodically telephoned into a center. Unobtrusive observers in the cafeteria determined food actually purchased and eaten. The telephoned and written food records had unacceptably high noncompliance rates, but they were slightly more accurate than the telephone recalls. "Evaluating the trade-offs between respondent burden, participation rates, and data accuracy, the study team concluded that 24-hour telephone recall, and the 7-day telephoned food record merited further investigation" (Shucker, 1982, p. 1308). One might question how generalizable these findings are, however, since this was nonrepresentative, college-age sample, and the subjects were aware of participating in a short term study, suggesting the possibility of confounding the results by measurement reactivity.

Although having unobtrusive observers watching people purchase and consume foods is an excellent technique for objectively determining food intake, in most situations it is not practical. However, biological markers of food or nutrient intake may prove to be useful. For example, Jacobson, Newmark, Bright-See, McKeown-Eyssen & Bruce (1983) have shown that the amount of 3-methylhistidine in a 24 hour urine sample correlates with the consumption of muscle meats on the previous day. Fecal fat is also directly associated with fat intake, except when diarrhea is present (Walker, Kelleher, Davies, Smith, & Losowsky, 1973) and fecal total weight, water, cellulose, or hemicellulose content may reflect total fiber intake (Wrick, Robertson, Van Soest, Lewis, Rivers, Roe, & Hackler, 1983). Hopefully, other such markers will be found, even if only reflecting recent food intake. These will be sufficient for the purpose of intervention trials. However, for population or case control studies, where the objective is to identify dietary factors which should be tested in clinical trials, markers of long term consumption of particular foods and/or nutrients will be needed.

Planning Dietary Trials in Cancer Prevention

In healthy populations at risk for a particular type of cancer, the objective is to change one or more components (e.g., nutrient, nonnutrient, additive, contaminant, specific food type) of the diet, preferably without altering total energy intake. In the study of healthy subjects, special information is needed prior to starting a clinical trial. What is the target population? What are the food habits of that group? Which of these habits are susceptible to modification either by manipulation or by education? The more information one has about the eating habits, cultural aversions and taboos, and eating motives of the study population, the easier it is to plan an effective clinical intervention.

Recent surveys of eating habits of Americans (Cronin, Krebs-Smith, Wyse, & Light, 1982) and Canadians (Health and Welfare Canada, 1973) are useful in describing in a broad way the general habits of specific segments of the population. For example, people over 51 years of age are more likely to eat crackers and cooked cereals and less likely to eat pasta and sandwiches than younger people. Women are more likely to eat yogurt and drink low calorie soft drinks than men (Cronin, et al., 1982). Another study (Meiselman & Wyant, 1981) found that males preferred beer, eggs, breakfast meats, meats, stews, and pies more than women, while women preferred appetizers, potatoes, potato substitutes, green vegetables, other vegetables, vegetable salads, tossed green salads and fresh fruit more than males. Such information is not sufficient for designing an intervention trial, but will help avoid planning an intervention around a food or type of food that is not acceptable to the majority of the study population. Such data are also useful in getting an overview of eating habits when a comprehensive dietary modification is planned.

Other sources of valuable information are marketing surveys, such as that conducted by the Market Research Corporation (Stowell, 1979). When data were compared to those from a 1972–1973 study, trends in food usage could be identified. The major finding was the continued decline in the proportion of foods eaten at home. Home use of wine, juices, poultry, salads, pasta and rice, as well as Italian, Mexican and Oriental dishes increased, while use of milk, coffee, total meat, fish, bread and sweetened or hot cereals decreased. In some instances the decreases for in-home consumption were offset by increased consumption away from home. For example, the use of all types of meats (except processed meats) and eggs increased in away-from-home usage. On the other hand, use of milk and coffee away from home also declined.

Determinants of the acceptance of particular foods have received more attention in recent years as the association between dietary variables and specific diseases of western civilization have been identified. Several models have been proposed to help explain the complex relationship between an individual and the foods he/she will or will not consume and the frequency of use of "acceptable" foods. For example, Rozin and Fallon (1981) suggested that the initial acceptance or rejection of a food is based on psychological categorization of three types: (1) the sensory-affective aspect of the food (i.e., taste and odor); (2) the anticipated consequence on either short-term or long-term physiological or social well being; and (3) idealized criteria of what is considered inappropriate or disgusting food in any culture.

Krondl and Law (1982) have proposed a model of social determinants in human food selection. Their model takes into account the cultural, economic and genetic aspects discussed by others. It also attempts to classify the various perceptions an individual may have of any one food or type of food. These include: satiety, tolerance, taste, familiarity, prestige, price, convenience, belief, and knowledge (the last two concerned with "healthfulness" of the food). These types of perceptions were tested in relation to the frequency of use of specific foods by a series of defined populations. In the Canadian groups studied, price, prestige and convenience of foods were found to be less important in influencing food consumption than either health belief or flavor of foods. Taste was the primary determinant for all age groups studied (adolescents, middle aged adult and elderly adults), but health belief became increasingly important in the older groups.

Studies of food consumption and models of eating behavior do not give the final answer in designing intervention trials. But as stated earlier, they do give clues to what would or would not be acceptable to a given population. If the intervention is to be based on education and motivation rather than manipulation of the food supply, additional efforts will be needed to tailor the intervention to the needs of the individual or subculture. For example, dieting (i.e., calorie restriction) is very common in Western culture. Weight fluctuation and chronic concern over caloric intake should be considered in the area of diet modification and cancer control.

Modifying Dietary Behavior in Trials

The purpose of a randomized dietary intervention trial is to study the relationship between diet and disease, in this case, cancer. To study this relationship, a strategy must be devised to systematically alter the diet of a defined population in such a way that compliance will be high and can be monitored, and only the factor(s) of interest will be changed, i.e., there is little if any disruption of other dietary components. Ethically, because these study populations are typically healthy, there must be few, if any, adverse side effects. It must also be possible, both technically and ethically, to arrange for an appropriate control group, taking particularly into account compliance and side effect issues.

Compliance in such trials clearly depends on the initial acceptability of the dietary intervention strategy and, more importantly, the ease with which dietary change can be incorporated into the subjects' lives for rather long periods of time. Again, designing such interventions requires a thorough knowledge of the eating patterns of the target population and the factors which determine these eating habits. The type of compliance monitoring that is feasible (for example, plasma monitoring or self-report telephone checks) will depend on the length of the study, the nature of the subjects, and the intervention itself.

Limiting disruption of dietary components other than the intervention target is important for two reasons. First, acceptance of and compliance with the regimen is likely to be greater with minimal disruption of the subject's eating and other habits. Second, alterations in aspects of the diet, other than the factor(s) under study, would confound interpretation of the results. Such confounding of dietary alterations would not be so critical in a management trial, i.e., where the primary purpose is to demonstrate a health effect rather than to define the mechanism of that response; however, dietary side effects should still be monitored if at all possible.

In designing dietary studies, as much care must go into planning for the control group as for the treatment group in order to be able to interpret validly any effects observed. Special placebo products or diets may need to be designed. In the case of overall diet, one must consider the ethics of recommending the *status quo* when recommendations from various health organizations (Note 1) suggest that changes might be appropriate. In order to facilitate compliance, the control subjects must believe that they are an important part of the study. A usual practice is to refrain from referring to the groups in the studies as "control" and "treatment" groups, but rather to refer to them as two different types of diet groups.

Decreasing Microcomponents. One's diet can be divided into microcomponents and macrocomponents. Examples of microcomponents are minerals, vitamins, or cooking byproduct components, whereas common macrocomponents include fat content, fiber content, and other major food components. Most people view the diet-cancer relationship as primarily causal and due to the presence of harmful "chemicals" in the diet (Whelan, 1980). Indeed there are some known carcinogens in the foods (Ames, 1983). While the exact contribution of such substances to human cancer incidence is not known, it is certainly desirable to ensure that their levels are minimized. The aim of food toxicological analysis is to modify the food supply at the production, handling and/or processing stages to ensure that as little as possible of these materials are present in food consumed by humans. For example, efforts are now being made to reduce the levels of nitrosamines and/or their precursors in foods by changing the processing of beer (Newmark & Mergens, 1981), lowering nitrates and nitrite levels in cured foods (Rice & Pierson, 1982) and adding inhibitors such as Vitamin C and Vitamin E (Newmark & Mergens, 1981) to block exogenous nitrosation in the foods.

It is doubtful that a randomized trial of this type of dietary modification, i.e., a trial testing the effect of toxic reduction, will ever be undertaken. By law in the United States any substance known to be carcinogenic must be removed from the food supply without any demonstration that the level of exposure constitutes a risk to human health. In contrast, epidemiological studies can demonstrate carcinogen-human cancer relationships. For example, the effect of a reduction on aflatoxin exposure on cancer rates in one part of a country heavily dependent in ground nuts and/or corn could be compared to cancer rates in an "untreated" area over an extended period of time. But again, an experimental trial with humans would be considered both unethical and illegal.

Increasing Microcomponents. The aim of studying increased levels of dietary microcomponents has been primarily that of chemoprevention or the study of nutritional pharmacology. The latter has been described as the "use of food components or derivatives thereof to achieve a pharmacological rather than a nutritional effect" (Spiller, 1981). Often the amounts of microcomponents used exceed amounts that could reasonably be consumed by the ingestion of food alone.

In recent years, vitamins and minerals (such as Vitamin A, carotene and retinoid derivatives, Vitamins C and E and selenium) have received particular attention. Intervention trials with such microfactors may be relatively easy in that compliance in the use of supplements should be more easily obtained than compliance with complex modification of the whole diet. Also, placebo capsules or tablets are not difficult to formulate, and therefore randomized blind trials are fairly easy to carry out.

The nutrient itself may serve as a compliance marker. For example, in a study we are currently conducting on Vitamins C and E, the Vitamin C content of the first urine sample of the morning is being used as a compliance check. In other cases—for example, the fat soluble vitamins which do not appear rapidly in the urine—a compliance marker could be added to the pill or capsule. One possible marker is riboflavin; its use is discussed later. Urine markers could also be used for checking the compliance of the placebo group.

In most intervention trials of micronutrients, the amounts given are much higher than what one could reasonably be expected to ingest from food. Thus, monitoring dietary intakes throughout the study may not be required. However, monitoring the use of nutrient supplements other than those prescribed by the trial is critical. General supplement use in North America is widespread and two of the vitamins of interest (C and E) are among the most widely used supplements. The potential for toxicity by ingesting large amounts of fatsoluble vitamins and trace minerals is well known and must be considered in their use. In the case of retinol or preformed Vitamin A, less toxic derivatives have been prepared (Sporn & Newton, 1979).

Decreasing Macrocomponents. Manipulation of macrocomponents is more difficult than altering microcomponents. Problems associated with disruption of usual eating practices, both for the individuals and their families, may hinder compliance. Also, alterations of ingested amounts of one macronutrient may affect consumption of other dietary components.

Boyd and his colleagues (this volume) described a study in which the fat intake of women with breast dysplasia is being reduced to about half of that of the usual North American diet. Compliance, as checked by fat intake calculated from food records and serum cholesterol values, has been acceptable, probably due to the intensive patient contacts and educational efforts made by these investigators. The maintenance of normal fat intake in the control group is also being monitored by dietary records and directly measured by serum cholesterol. Data indicate that fecal fat may also serve as a compliance marker for low fat diets (Walker et al., 1973). The use of this measure is being investigated in a subsample of this test population. A preliminary test showed a minor increase in fiber intake in the low fat diet group (unpublished results). A major difficulty has been the unwillingness or inability of some women to replace the energy lost from decreased fat intake by increased carbohydrate intake. Thus, maintenance of body weight has been a problem with some subjects.

The control group in this study is being counseled to follow a diet as recommended by *Canada's Food Guide* (Health Promotion Directorate, 1982). This approach to a placebo may not be feasible in the future as the *Guide* has now been revised to include a recommendation to "decrease your total fat intake."

Increasing Macrocomponents. The major macro-factor of current interest in cancer research is dietary fiber, or more precisely, dietary fibers, as several substances of diverse chemical composition are classed as fibers (Southgate, 1979). A high fiber snack (HFS), supplying approximately 20 grams of dietary fiber from wheat bran per daily intake, and low fiber snack (LFS), with about 3.5 grams of fiber per daily intake, have been prepared as tools for a study of the effect of dietary fiber on the recurrence of adenomatous polyps of the colon. These products were tested for acceptability, side-effects, and effects on other dietary variables in a small group of healthy adults (Bright-See, McKeown-Eyssen, Jacobson, Newark, Mathews, Morison, & Bruce, in preparation).

Compliance was checked by daily records kept by the subjects and by periodic check of riboflavin in 24-hour urine samples (riboflavin was added to both snack products as a marker). Urinary riboflavin output was variable depending on the amount and timing of snacks eaten. In a few cases, unusually high initial values were found due to supplement use. Also, urinary riboflavin represented only periodic checks and may or may not have reflected "usual" consumption of the snacks. On the other hand, records relied on the memory and the honesty of the subjects. The combination of the two methods helped identify subjects who were probably not complying, i.e., those who reported low intakes and/or consistently had low urinary riboflavin values. The compliance rate, as assessed by these methods, was quite acceptable. Wet stool weights as well as total fecal hemicellulose and cellulose were greater when the HFS, rather than the LFS, was consumed. These parameters are being studied as possible markers of total dietary fiber intake.

Overall, dietary changes were followed by 4-day food records kept at the beginning, middle, and end of the study. Consumption of the snacks caused no significant change in the voluntary intake (i.e., not including the snack) of energy, protein, fat, carbohydrate, calcium, iron, Vitamin A, Vitamin C, thiamin, riboflavin and niacin. Use of HFS did cause a reduction in voluntary dietary fiber consumption of about 3.1 grams a day.

Several health parameters were also monitored. Body weights, blood pressure, and hemoglobin values remained within normal limits for most subjects. However, mean serum ferritin values tended to decrease over the study period with both LFS and HFS, and three of the 28 subjects had values below the accepted normal range (18 grams/liter) at the end of the study. Most serum calcium values were in the low normal range (below 9.5 milligrams/decaliter), and five subjects had values below 8.5 mg/dl at some time during the study. Thus, for the long term intervention, the snacks products will be enriched with iron and calcium. In addition, serum and hair copper, zinc and magnesium will be checked periodically to detect any possible effect of the intervention on the status of these trace elements. Such findings reemphasize the need for preliminary testing of any proposed intervention tool or system.

Multiple Factor Intervention. Interventions using several dietary factors may be unavoidable because it is unrealistic to alter one dietary variable without changing others. Also, such studies may be necessary because restrictions in time or number of subjects do not allow for the independent testing of each dietary variable. Two frequently associated dietary factors are fat and fibers, low fiber and high fat availability being strongly associated with colon cancer mortality (McKeown-Eyssen & Bright-See, 1982). The ability and willingness of women to adhere to a low fat diet (Boyd et al., this volume), as well as the ability of a group of men and women to consume supplemental fiber (McKeown-Eyssen & Bright-See, 1982), have been demonstrated. Compliance to a double fiber–fat intervention was studied in a small group of men (Note 4). Reported total snack intake was over 85% for four of the five subjects. Twenty four hour urinary riboflavin output and 24-hour fecal wet weights also indicated appreciable fiber consumption in these four subjects. Fat intakes were calculated at the beginning and three times during the study. The initial fat intake was about 35% of total energy. This dropped to 21 to 25% of total energy over the two month study time.

As indicated earlier, in a current fat reduction intervention trial by Boyd et al. (this volume), maintenance of total energy intake was a problem as some women failed to replace the energy from fat-containing foods with carbohydrates. In the preliminary fiber trial, there was some indication that subjects were not compensating for the energy in the snacks by decreasing their voluntary energy intake. In the combined fiber/fat intervention, the average total energy intake (voluntary plus snack) was the same at one and two months as at the beginning of the study. In the trial of fiber alone, ingestion of the HFS led to a decrease in voluntary fiber intake. That did not occur when the HFS was accompanied by a low fat diet. Thus, these two interventions appear to be complementary and therefore adherence to both in a long-term trial may be better than adherence to either dietary modification alone.

Interventions in the Current North American Environment

It is often said that it is difficult to get people to change how they eat (Beidler, 1982). However, eating habits of North Americans are changing (Stowell, 1979; Health Promotion Directorate, 1979; Grocery Products Manufacturers of Canada, 1980). Much of this change can be attributed to the current interest in nutrition initiated by the many dietary recommendations made to the public (Department of National Health and Welfare, 1980) and promoted both by governments and food industries. This atmosphere is both advantageous and disadvantageous to many of the intervention studies either underway or being considered. For example, nutrient supplement use is wide-spread so it is at least potentially easy to convince subjects to take "pills" as prescribed. On the other hand, comparison must be monitored carefully as doses of some nutrients (e.g., Vitamins C and E) in commercially available preparations equal or exceed the treatment doses (Enstrom & Pauling, 1982).

The increasing availability of high fiber and low fat products makes adherence to a high fiber–low fat intervention more likely. Even with the current emphasis on this two dietary-factor ingestion, it is unlikely that voluntary intake of control groups will reach the treatment levels of experimental groups (50 grams fat and 45 grams of dietary fiber) within the near future. Extrapolating from the data cited by Stamler (1982), and assuming a 3000 Kcal daily intake for men and a 2000 kilocalories daily intake for women, the average daily fat intake will reach 50 grams per day around the year 2000 *if* the current downward trend continues. The interest in dietary fiber is fairly recent (since Burkitt, 1973), and there is no documentation of how this interest may affect total fiber intake.

Recent experience in clinical trials of dietary and other risk factors for cardiovascular disease (Zukel, Paul, & Schnaper, 1981) illustrated that while it is possible to demonstrate that the treatment group responded appropriately to an effective intervention, changes in the habits of the control group can account for a failure to demonstrate significant differences in cardiovascular mortality between the two groups. That is, due to nonplanned dietary and other lifestyle changes occurring in society at large, end results may blur between the treatment and "control" groups. Thus, it is necessary to try to predict what changes in the factors of interest may reasonably be expected to occur in the control group over the time of the study.

In summary, a clear definition of the dietary factor(s) to be changed and a thorough understanding of the study population and their eating habits and motives will be necessary in any experimental test of diet effect on disease risk. Ingenious methods of altering dietary factors can be devised given the current technological status and cooperative interest of the food and pharmaceutical industries. For example, technologies such as clever placebo packaging and markers of experimental "doses" may prove effective and practical. In terms of feasibility and cost-effectiveness, we need to know the *least* intensive intervention strategy necessary to achieve dietary change. A treatment package found to be valid for clinical change in an individual patient may not be feasible in a trial involving 5000 subjects over a five-year duration.

DIET AND CANCER

Food Consumption in Patient Populations

In the study of diet and cancer, the issue is not control of total food intake. Rather, in cancer patients, the major concern is usually how to increase total energy and nutrient intake in order to override factors repressing food consumption. The eating behavior and consequent nutritional status of cancer patients can be viewed as a function of tumor burden or as a function of treatment side effects, such as nausea during a chemotherapy course. For example, in one study (Donaldson, 1982), overt malnutrition was seen in 17% of children with newly diagnosed localized tumors, and in 37% of patients with metastatic disease. In a second retrospective study of 1000 patients with a variety of neoplastic disorders, significant weight loss occurred in nearly half the sample (Costa and Donaldson, 1980). Although it is recognized that all weight loss in cancer patients is not simply a function of lowered caloric intake, eating difficulties contribute significantly to cachexic status (Bernstein, 1982).

The development of nutritional deficit is also not simply related to extent of tumor burden, anatomical site involved, or cell type. Neither is degree of physical wasting directly associated with the anatomical involvement of the tumor. Attempts have been made to identify metabolic effects of cancer cells, but except for a few ectopic hormones (Odell and Wolfsen, 1978), no tumor "toxin" has been thus far unequivocably identified (Costa and Donaldson, 1980).

As DeWys discusses in this volume, patient weight loss is generally attributable to a "negative energy balance", because of decreased caloric intake, coupled with altered and increased energy expenditure by the host

> . . . alterations in protein metabolism include preferential uptake of amino acids by the tumor, decreased synthesis of some host tissue proteins such as muscle tissue, and increased synthesis of other host proteins. Lipid metabolism is seemingly less affected. These metabolic changes result in muscle wasting in adult cancer patients and growth failure in pediatric cancer patients. Host tissues are catabolized to meet the nutritional demands of the tumor, and nutritional death may ensue. (DeWys, 1982, p. 721).

Ultimately, the pathological limiting factor is not the patient's nutritional status, but the biology of the tumor invading the host (Levine, Brennan, Ramu, Fisher, Pizzo, & Glavbiger, 1982).

In addition to metabolic effects of neoplasia, caloric intake is frequently reduced by nausea, vomiting and loss of appetite in patients under treatment. These side effects of toxic therapies are sometimes themselves learned behavioral phenomena associated with the treatment context (Bernstein, 1982). Morrow (1982) has reported that approximately 21% of cancer patients in his study experienced learned or "anticipatory" nausea and vomiting before chemotherapy treatment. Bernstein and Webster, Redd, Burish, and Andrykowski, and Burish, Redd, and Carey discuss these associative side effects at length in this volume.

Dietary Intervention in Patient Populations

In patient populations, the challenge of dietary intervention is heightened by the effects of tumor burden and toxic regimens. As Levine points out in his chapter in this volume, a limiting factor in cancer treatment is not necessarily the patient's nutritional status, but rather may be the biology of the tumor process. Still, the side effects of aggressive treatment affect patient stamina and biological vulnerability, and the control of eating in patient populations is very important.

Redd, Burish, & Andrykowski (this volume) describe in detail their specific techniques to counter nausea and vomiting, capitalizing on learning principles, as well as utilizing the relaxation response with its associated biological correlates (Hoffman, Benson, Arns, Stainbrook, Landsberg, Young, & Gill, 1982). Grunberg (this volume) also suggests capitalizing on the possibility of particular food preferences within patient groups, assessing and utilizing these preferences for research purposes in order to uncover possible mechanisms of weight change in patient groups. He also points out that for treatment purposes, such shifts in preference can be utilized in menu preparation in order to maintain or enhance nutritional status.

There are other kinds of ancillary behavioral techniques that can be used in the service of patient nutritional support. For example, Costa and Donaldson (1980) discussed the use of behavioral modification techniques such as behavioral shaping and cognitive preparation in support of dietary, mechanical interventions such as tube feeding.

RESEARCH AND TRAINING PRIORITIES

Potentially effective clinical techniques for diet modification are now available for use in community and patient settings. Techniques such as cognitive preparation, relaxation and hypnosis, counter-conditioning in the treatment of food aversions, and so on are all examples of intervention strategies that have proven moderately effective in individual and small group samples (Stunkard & Penick, 1979). Whether they are equally effective or even feasible in a large scale clinical trial is still an empirical question.

In terms of research training—particularly at the postdoctoral level—behavioral scientists need to be trained in clinical trial and epidemiological methodology as well as the nutritional and practical aspects of foods and food usage. They also need to have research training in oncology in order to know the biological disease as it is potentially affected by dietary intervention. As in any behavioral medicine endeavor, one cannot ask questions relevant to the end-points of a disease without having a firm grasp of its biological base. In turn, oncologists and epidemiologists need to learn the language of behavioral science, and begin to collaborate with behavioral and social scientists in all phases of research planning and conduct. In fact, these disciplines can contribute across all stages of trial intervention. In the planning phases of an intervention trial, behavioral issues associated with the cost (labor intensity required to induce and maintain adherence to protocol, for example) need to be taken into account in estimating sample size and budget needs. In the recruitment phase, behavioral issues related to informed consent, recruitment of high risk subjects, and trial induction need to be considered. During the whole phase of trial intervention, as well as during trial closure, other issues such as staff training in adherence methods, subject debriefing, and interpretation of trial results related to compliance level and subgroup compliance distribution require behavioral science expertise. In short, continued theoretical and clinical advances in the area of diet and cancer may increasingly depend on the cross fertilization between behavioral science and oncology.

REFERENCES

Ackerman, L. V., Weinstein, I. B., & Kaplan, H. S. (1978). Cancer of the esophagus. In H. S. Kaplan & P. J. Tsuchitani (Eds.), *Cancer in China*. New York: Alan R. Liss, Inc.

Ames, B. N. (1983). Dietary carcinogens and anticarcinogens. *Science, 221*, 1256–1264.

Beidler, L. M. (1982). Biological bases of food selection. In L. M. Barker (Ed.), *The psychobiology of human food selection.* Westport, CT: AVI Publishing Company, Inc.

Bernstein, I. (1982). Physiological and psychological mechanisms of cancer anorexia. *Cancer Research, 42,* 715–719.

Block, G. (1982). A review of validations of dietary assessment methods. *American Journal of Epidemiology, 115,* 492–505.

Bright-See, E., McKeown-Eyssen, G. E., Jacobson, E. A., Newark, H. C., Mathews, R., Morison, L., & Bruce, W. R. *Evaluation of a tool for the study of dietary fiber.* In preparation.

Brownell, K. (1982). Obesity: Understanding and treating a serious, prevalent, and refractory disorder. *Journal of Community and Clinical Psychology, 50,* 820–840.

Burkitt, D. P. (1973). Some diseases characteristic of modern Western civilization. *British Medical Journal, 1,* 274–278.

Chlebowski, R., Heber, D., & Block, J. (1983). Lung cancer cachexia. In F. Greco (Ed.), *Biology and Management of Lung Cancer.* The Hague: Martinus Nijhoff.

Costa, G., & Donaldson, S. (1980). The nutritional effects of cancer and its therapy. *Nutrition and Cancer, 2,* 22–29.

Cronin, F. J., Krebs-Smith, S. M., Wyse, B. W., & Light, L. (1982). Characterizing food usage by demographic variables. *Journal of American Dietary Association, 81,* 661–673.

Department of National Health and Welfare. (1980) *Nutrition recommendations for Canadians,* Ottawa, Canada, 1980.

DeWys, W. (1982). Pathophysiology of cancer cachexia: current understanding and areas for future research. *Cancer Research, 42,* 721–725.

Doll, R., & Peto, R. (1981). The causes of cancer: qualitative estimates of avoidable risks of cancer in the United States today. *Journal of the National Cancer Institute, 66,* 1194–1265.

Donaldson, S. (1982). Effects of therapy on nutritional status of the pediatric patient. *Cancer Research, 42,* 729–734.

Enstrom, J. E., & Pauling, L. (1982). Mortality among health-conscious elderly Californians. *Proceedings of National Academy of Sciences U.S.A., 79,* 6023–6027.

Goodstein, R. (1983). *Eating and weight disorders.* New York: Springer.

Graham, S. (1980). Diet and cancer. *American Journal of Epidemiology, 112,* 247–252.

Grocery Products Manufacturers of Canada. (1979). *Food and nutrition survey report.* Toronto.

Health and Welfare Canada. (1973). *Nutrition Canada, national survey.* Ottawa.

Health Promotion Directorate, Health and Welfare Canada. (1982). *Canda's food guide (revised).* Ottawa.

Health Promotion Directorate, Health and Welfare Canada. (1979). *Report on nutrition concepts evaluation study.* Ottawa.

Hoffman, J., Benson, H., Arns, P., Stainbrook, G., Landsberg, L., Young, J., & Gill, A. (1982). Reduced sympathetic nervous system responsivity associated with the neoplastic response. *Science, 215,* 190–192.

Jacobson, E. A., Newmark, H. L., McKeown-Eyssen, G., Bruce, W. R. (1983). Excretion of 3-Methylhistidine in the urine as an estimate of meat consumption. *Nutrition Reports International, 27,* 1983.

Krantzler, N., Mullen, B., Comstock, E., Holden, C., Schultz, H., Brevetti, L., & Meiselman, H. (1982). Methods of food intake assessment—an annotated bibliography. *Journal Nutrition Education, 14,* 108–119.

Krondl, M., & Lau, D. (1982). Social determinants in human food selection. In L. N. Baker (Ed.), *The psychobiology of human food selection.* Westport, CT: AVI Publishing Co., Inc.

Levine, A., Brennan, M., Ramu, A., Fisher, R., Pizzo, P., & Glavbiger, D. (1982). Controlled clinical trials of nutritional intervention as an adjunct to chemotherapy, with a comment on nutrition and drug resistance. *Cancer Research, 42,* 774–778.

Madden, J., Goodman, S., & Guture, H. (1976). Validity of the 24-hour recall: Analysis of data obtained from elderly subjects. *Journal of the American Diet Association, 68,* 143–147.

Marshall, J., Priore, R., Haughey, B., Rzepka, T., & Graham, S. (1980). Spouse-subject interviews and the reliability of diet studies. *American Journal of Epidemiology, 112,* 675–683.

McKeown-Eyssen, G., & Bright-See, E. (1982). Relationship between colon cancer mortality and fibre availability: an international study. *International Symposium on Dietary Fiber,* New Zealand.

Meiselman, H. L., & Wyant, K. W. (1981). Food preferences and flavor experiences. In J. Solms & R. L. Hall (Eds.), *Criteria for food acceptance.* Zurich: Forster Publishing Ltd.

Morrow, G. (1982). Prevalence and correlates of anticipatory nausea and vomiting in chemotherapy patients. *Journal of the National Cancer Institute, 68,* 585–588.

Murphy, R., & Michael, G. (1982). Methodologic considerations of the National Health and Nutrition Examination Survey. *The American Journal of Clinical Nutrition, 35,* 1255–1258.

National Research Council (1982). Committee on Diet, Nutrition and Cancer. *Diet, nutrition and Cancer.* Washington, DC: National Academy press.

Newmark, H. L., & Mergens, W. J. (1981). Applications of ascorbic acid and tocopherals as inhibitors of nitrosamine formation and oxidation in foods. In J. Solms & R. L. Hall (Eds.), *Criteria for food acceptance.* Zurich: Forster Publishing Ltd.

Odell, W., & Wolfsen, A. (1978). Humoral syndromes associated with cancer. *Annual Review of Medicine, 29,* 379–406.

Rice, K. N., & Pierson, M. D. (1982). Inhibition of salmonella by sodium nitrate and potassium sorbate in frankfurters. *Journal of Food Science, 47,* 1615–1617.

Rozin, P., & Fallon, A. E. (1981). The acquisition of likes and dislikes for foods. In J. Solms & R. L. Hall (Eds.), *Criteria of food acceptance.* Zurich: Forster Publishing Ltd.

Segi, M. (1980). Age-adjusted death rates for cancer for selected sites (A-classification) in 46 countries in 1975. *Segi Institute of Cancer Epidemiology,* Nayoya, Japan.

Schucker, R. (1982). Alternative approaches to clinic food consumption measurement methods: Telephone interviewing and market data bases. *The American Journal of Clinical Nutrition, 35,* 1306–1309.

Southgate, D. A. T. (1979). The definition, analyses and properties of dietary fibre. In K. W. Heaton (Ed.), *Dietary fibre: Current developments of importance to health.* Westport, CT: Technomic Publishing Co., Inc.

Spiller, G. A. (1981). *Current Topics in Nutrition and Disease, 4,* 1.

Spitzer, L., & Rodin, J. (1981). Human eating behavior: A critical review of studies in normal weight and overweight individuals. *Appetite: Journal for Intake Research, 2,* 293–329.

Sporn, M. B., & Newton, D. L. (1979). Chemoprevention of cancer with retinoids. *Proceedings of Federal American Society for Experimental Biology, 38,* 2528–2534.

Stamler, J. (1982). Diet and coronary heart disease. *Biometrics, 38* Suppl., 195–214.

Stowell, C. (1979 December). Marketers to fight for declining in-home sector as food consumption patterns change. *Food Product Developments,* pp. 95–97.

Stunkard, A., & Penick, S. (1979). Behavior modification in the treatment of obesity: The problem of maintaining weight loss. *Archives of Behavioral Psychiatry, 36,* 801–802.

Stunkard, A., & Waxman, M. (1981). Accuracy of self reports of food intake. *Journal of the American Dietetic Association, 79,* 547–551.

Walker, B. E., Kelleher, J., Davies, T., Smith, C. L., & Losowsky, M. S. (1973). Influence of dietary fat on fecal fat. *Gastroenterology, 64,* 233–239.

Whelan, E. (1980). *Preventing cancer.* New York: W. W. Norton & Company.

Wrick, K. L., Robertson, J. B., Van Soest, P. J., Lewis, B. A., Rivers, J. M., Roe, D. A., & Hackler, L. R. (1983). The influence of dietary fibre source on human intestinal transit and stool output. *Journal of Nutrition, 113,* 1464–1479.

Zukel, W., Paul, O., & Schnaper, H. (1981). The multiple risk factor intervention trial (MRFIT). *Preventive Medicine, 10,* 387–400.

10 Diet and Breast Disease: Evidence for the Feasibility of a Clinical Trial Involving a Major Reduction in Dietary Fat

N. F. Boyd, M.B., B.S.
Ontario Cancer Institute; Ludwig Institute for Cancer Research, Toronto

M. L. Cousins
S. E. Bayliss
Ludwig Institute for Cancer Research, Toronto

E. B. Fish, M.D.
E. Fishnell, M. B.
Women's College Hospital

W. R. Bruce, M.D.
Ludwig Institute for Cancer Research, Toronto

INTRODUCTION

Breast cancer is the most common neoplasm affecting women in the Western World (Doll, Muir, & Waterhouse, 1976), and a substantial proportion of women who develop the disease will ultimately die of it (Mueller & Jeffries, 1975). It is estimated that each year in the United States, 100,000 new cases of breast cancer are diagnosed, and that there are 30,000 deaths from the disease (Kelsey, 1979). Mortality from breast cancer has not changed over a prolonged period of time and shows no evidence of having been improved substantially by improvements in surgical care (Armstrong, 1976; Devesa & Silverman, 1978). Although it is possible that recent developments in adjuvant therapy may reduce mortality from breast cancer, the existing data suggest that any influence of the presently available treatments is likely to be small (Rossi, Bonnadonna, Valagussa, & Veronesi, 1981; Fisher, Redmond, Brown, Wolmark, Wittliff, Fisher, Plotkin, Bowman, Sachs, Wolter, Geggie, Campbell, Elias, Prager, Koontz, Volk, Kimitroy, Gardner, Lerner, & Shibata, 1981).

In the absence of any potent new therapy for breast cancer, there appear to be two major approaches to reducing the impact of the disease. One approach is concerned with early detection through screening, and is supported by evidence from a randomized controlled trial showing that mortality from breast cancer can be reduced in women over the age of 50 by annual screening with physical examination and mammography (Shapiro, 1977). Evidence of a benefit from screening in younger women, in terms of reduced mortality from breast cancer, is not presently available, but is now being sought in a further randomized controlled trial of screening (Miller, Howe & Wall, 1981). However, screening populations with mammography is an expensive undertaking, and there is concern about the hazards of exposing breast tissue to ionizing radiation (Bailar, 1977).

A second possible approach to the problem would be to devise methods of prevention. The evidence that breast cancer, and other common malignancies, may be preventable has recently been reviewed by Doll and Peto (1981) and is derived from epidemiologic observations that show a striking international variation in breast cancer incidence and mortality. Breast cancer incidence and mortality are generally low in far Eastern and African countries, and high in North America and Europe (Doll, Muir, & Waterhouse, 1976). The variation in breast cancer incidence may be as great as seven-fold, as it is for example, between North America and Japan or the non-Jewish inhabitants of Israel, and is influenced by age. Breast cancer in women under the age of 50 is approximately four times more common in North America than in Japan, but after that age there is an approximately eight-fold difference in the incidence of the disease between these countries.

Studies of migrants provide evidence that these international differences in breast cancer incidence are not due to genetic factors, but rather are attributable to environmental influences. Migrants moving from countries of low breast cancer incidence to high incidence countries eventually acquire the breast cancer incidence of the country to which they move (Buell, 1973, Haenszel and Kurihara, 1968), a change that may take two or three generations. The similar breast cancer incidence rates experienced by Japanese and Caucasian inhabitants of Hawaii, both of which are substantially greater than the rates of Japanese living in Japan, provide a particularly good example of this phenomenon (Doll, Muir, & Waterhouse, 1976). Changes observed in breast cancer incidence within countries provide further evidence for an environmental influence. Such changes have, for example, been observed recently in Iceland (Bjarnason, Day, & Snaedal & Tulinius, 1974) and Japan (Hirayama, 1979).

Evidence Relating Diet and Breast Cancer

Although these observations suggest that breast cancer incidence may be related to environmental factors, they do not indicate which of the many environmental differences between countries is responsible. There is, however, considerable circumstantial evidence indicating that diet may play a role in the etiology of breast cancer.

The evidence relating diet and breast cancer risk has been the subject of recent reviews (Reddy, Cohen, McCoy, Hill, Weisburger, & Wynder, 1980; Carroll, Gammel, & Plunkett, 1968; Miller, 1977). Several workers have shown that the international variation in breast cancer incidence is strongly correlated with estimates of per capita fat consumption (Reddy et al, 1980; Carroll et al, 1968; Armstrong & Doll, 1975; Lea, 1966; Draser & Irving, 1973), and this association appears to be strongest for fats of animal rather than vegetable origin.

Analysis of changes in breast cancer incidence within countries also shows a positive correlation with changes in dietary fat consumption. For example, the rise in breast cancer incidence observed in Japan since 1950 has occurred at the same time as the adoption of a more Western style of life, including increased consumption of meat, eggs, and milk products (Hirayama, 1979). Within the United States, Seventh Day Adventists have lower breast mortality and lower dietary fat consumption than the rest of the population (Phillips, 1975).

Case control studies within countries have shown a relatively weak (Miller, 1978) or absent (Graham et al., 1982) relationship between fat intake and breast cancer risk. It is not at present clear to what extent these results are due to the acknowledged difficulty in obtaining information about lifelong dietary practices, the lack of variation in dietary habits within populations, or a genuinely weak association.

These epidemiologic observations of a relationship between fat intake and breast cancer incidence in human populations derive considerable support from experimental studies with animals. Tannenbaum and Silverstone (1957) have shown that the formation of mammary tumors in mice is promoted by obesity and retarded by caloric restriction, and that isocaloric diets high and low in fat are associated respectively with a high and low incidence of mammary tumors (Tannenbaum 1942). In studies with chemically induced mammary tumors in mice Carroll and Khor (1975) have shown that dietary fat increases tumor formation only when given after tumor initiation, indicating that in this system dietary fat acts as a tumor promoter.

The mechanism by which dietary fat might influence the development of breast cancer is unknown, but several metabolic alterations have been reported in association with changes in fat consumption that might influence the state of the mammary epithelium. Mammary epithelial cells are sensitive to the actions of several hormones, including prolactin, estrogen, progesterone, glucocorticoid, insulin and growth hormone (Toppler & Freeman, 1980). Plasma levels of prolactin and estrogen have been shown by some to be influenced by the diet consumed (Hill & Wynder, 1976) but not by others (Gray, Pike, & Henderson, 1981). Levels of insulin and growth hormone are also influenced by dietary factors (Williams, 1968). Although the relevance of changes in these hormones to human mammary carcinogenesis is presently unknown, they do provide one mechanism by which diet might influence the state of mammary epithelial cells. However, extensive investigations have, so far, failed to reveal any hormonal profile that is uniquely associated with breast cancer risk (Pike, Siiteri, & Welsch, 1981), and the possibility exists that dietary fat, or one of its products, may act directly upon mammary epithelial cells to promote tumor formation (Hopkins & West, 1976; Mukai & Goldstein, 1976).

Strategies for Dietary Intervention Studies in Breast Cancer

Hypotheses concerning the relationship of diet to breast cancer risk, generated by either epidemiological observations or animal experimentation, need to be tested in humans before we can be assured of their relevance to human disease. Dietary intervention studies, in which a dietary change is made in a group of individuals who are then observed for a change in the frequency of cancer, are an attractively direct way of testing such hypotheses. Studies of this type, however, pose formidable methodological difficulties. These include the relative infrequency of even the most common human tumors, and in consequence, the long periods of observation and large sample sizes required to detect an effect of dietary change upon cancer incidence. Additional difficulties arise from the need to bring about a change in the dietary practices of free-living human populations, while maintaining a control group that does not change its dietary habits; and the need to maintain and follow these groups over an extended period of time.

An alternative strategy that allows at least some of these problems to be circumvented is to use a change in a lesion that is a precursor to cancer, rather than cancer itself, as the target measure for dietary intervention studies (Bruce, Eyssen, Ciampi, Dion, & Boyd, 1981). Because precursor lesions can generally be expected to be much more common events than deaths from even the most common tumors, the use of a precursor to cancer as a target measure for dietary intervention may allow much smaller sample sizes and shorter periods of follow-up than would be required if death from cancer were the target. It is also methodologically more straightforward to determine whether a lesion has been reversed than to demonstrate that an event, such as death from cancer, has been prevented. This strategy, of course, requires that precursors be identified that are early stages in the development of cancer, and that reversal or prevention of the precursor lesions could be expected to lead to a reduction in the frequency of cancer.

To apply this strategy to breast cancer it is first necessary to identify a risk factor that is a suitable target for dietary intervention. None of the many well-documented risk factors for breast cancer, such as parity, age at first pregnancy, or family history of breast cancer, is susceptible to change in affected individuals. To examine the effect of nutrition on breast cancer risk we first examined evidence that the breast itself, as assessed by mammography, contained information about risk.

Mammographic Signs as Risk Factors for Breast Cancer

Wolfe has described a method of classifying the appearance of the breast parenchyma as seen in mammography in a way that purportedly allows us to identify groups with substantially different risks for the subsequent development of breast cancer (Wolfe, 1976; Wolfe, Albert, Belle & Sulane, 1982). In this system of classification the mammographic appearance associated with the lowest risk of breast cancer, designated "N", is characterized by a breast comprised almost exclusively of fat and connective tissue. Two categories associated with different degrees of intermediate risk are distinguished by the extent of ductal prominence. In the lower risk category, "P1", prominent ducts occupy less than 25% of the breast volume. In "P2", the higher risk category, prominent ducts occupy 25% or more of the breast volume. The category designated "DY" is associated with the highest risk of breast cancer and is defined as "severe mammary dysplasia."

A number of other studies have shown these categories to be associated with different risks for the development of breast cancer (Krook, Carlile, Bush & Hall, 1978; Krook, 1975; Threatt, Norbeck, Ullman, Kummer, & Rosell, 1980; Wilkinson, Clopton, Gordonson, Green, Hill, & Pike, 1977; Hainline, Myers, McLelland, Newell, Grufferman, & Shingleton, 1978; Brisson, Sadowsky, Twaddle, Morrison, Cole, & Merletti, 1982; Chaudary, Gravelle, Bulstrode, Wana, Millis, & Hayward, 1983; Boyd, O'Sullivan, Campbell, Fishell, Simor, Cooke, & Germanson, 1982a; Boyd et al., 1982b) and have, in general, confirmed that the DY category is associated with the highest risk. However, not all studies have shown this relationship (Mendell, Rosenbloom & Naimark, 1977; Rideout & Poon, 1977; Ernster, Sack, Peterson, & Schweitzer, 1980; Moskowitz, Gartside, & McLaughlin, 1980), and the subject is still widely regarded as controversial. It appears, however, that the contradictory results that have given rise to this controversy arise at least in part from the failure of some studies to observe the usual methodologic standards employed in epidemiologic research (Boyd, O'Sullivan, Fishell, Simor, & Cooke, 1984).

To examine the association between mammographic signs and breast cancer, we carried out a case control study in which 183 women with breast cancer ("cases") and 183 women without breast cancer ("controls") were matched by age to form case control pairs (Boyd et al., 1982b). The cases and controls all had mammograms performed in the Department of Radiology at Women's College Hospital. The controls were selected from women who had volunteered for a feasibility study of breast cancer screening and were free of any breast abnormality thought to require diagnostic evaluation. The cases had histologically verified unilateral breast cancer. Mammograms from the noncancerous breast of the cases and from the corresponding breast of the controls were randomly mixed, and independently classified by three radiologists who were unaware of which mammograms were from cases and which were from controls. Data on the bilateral symmetry of mammographic patterns are presented elsewhere (Boyd et al., 1982).

The three radiologists each classified the proportion of breast volume occupied by the changes of ductal prominence and dysplasia, and classified the mammogram according to Wolfe's nomenclature.

The relationship between the proportion of the breast occupied by dysplasia and breast cancer is shown in Table 10.1. In general, dysplasia was more common among cases than controls, particularly the most extensive category in which 75% or more of the breast volume contained dysplastic changes. Dysplasia occupying 75% or more of the breast was seen in 32 (17%) of the cases and only 7 (4%) of the controls according to Radiologist A. Radiologist C obtained similar results. Each radiologist found a statistically significant relationship between the most extensive category of dysplasia and breast cancer. A monotonic increment in this association from the localized to the more extensive categories of dysplasia was found only by Radiologist C.

Because the prevalence of mammary dysplasia is known to vary with age, we analyzed the association between breast cancer and dysplasia taking age into

TABLE 10.1
Distribution of Cases and Controls According to Extent of Dysplasis and Radiologist (all ages)

	Extent of Dysplasia[d]					
Radiologist	<10%	10<25%	25<50%	50<75%	<75%	Total
A						
Controls	139(76)	9(5)	14(8)	14(8)	7(4)	183
Cases	105(57)	13(7)	17(9)	16(9)	31(17)	183
Odds ratio	1.00	1.89	1.59	1.50	5.99[a]	
B						
Controls	103(56)	23(13)	24(13)	18(10)	15(8)	183
Cases	78(43)	32(17)	18(10)	22(12)	33(18)	183
Odds ratio	1.00	1.84	0.99	1.61	2.82[b]	
C						
Controls	140(77)	14(8)	12(7)	8(4)	9(5)	183
Cases	104(57)	12(7)	20(11)	22(12)	25(14)	183
Odds ratio	1.00	1.15	2.24	3.70	3.74[c]	

[a] x_2^2=18.96; p 0.0001
[b] x_2^2=8.99; p=0.002
[c] x^2=10.25; p=0.001
[d] % in parentheses

TABLE 10.2
Distribution of Cases and Controls According to Extent of Dysplasia and Radiologist (aged under 50)

Radiologist	Extent of Dysplasia[d] <10%	10<25%	25<50%	50<75%	>75%	Total
A						
Controls	56(70)	2(3)	8(10)	10(13)	4(5)	80
Cases	36(45)	6(8)	9(11)	10(13)	19(24)	80
Odds ratio	1.00	4.67	1.75	1.56	7.39[a]	
B						
Controls	36(45)	12(15)	14(18)	11(14)	7(9)	80
Cases	19(24)	18(23)	11(14)	14(18)	18(23)	80
Odds ratio	1.00	2.84	1.49	2.41	4.87[b]	
C						
Controls	57(71)	8(10)	5(6)	4(5)	6(8)	80
Cases	32(40)	8(10)	11(14)	12(15)	17(21)	80
Odds ratio	1.00	1.78	3.92	5.34	5.05[c]	

[a] $X^2=12.25; p=0.0002$
[b] $X^2=8.25; p=0.004$
[c] $X^2=9.21; p=0.002$
[d] % in parentheses

account. Table 10.2 shows the distribution of cases and controls, aged less than 50, according to the extent of dysplasia. Each radiologist again found that dysplasia occupied 75% or more of the breast volume more frequently among cases than among controls. Between 21% and 24% of the cases were placed in this category according to each of the radiologists, compared to between 5% and 9% of the controls. Each radiologist again found a statistically significant association between the most extensive category of dysplasia and breast cancer.

A significant relationship between dysplasia and breast cancer was not found among women over the age of 50, and dysplasia of any extent was less common among women over the age of 50 than it was among younger women. The proportion of the breast occupied by the radiologic changes of ductal prominence was not found to be consistently associated with breast cancer, and no association emerged after taking age into account in this analysis.

A comparison of Wolfe's classification with a classification based upon the extent of dysplasia showed that the extent of dysplasia discriminated more strongly between cases and controls. When the additional risk factors of age at first live birth, parity, and family history of breast cancer were included in the analysis, the association between dysplasia and breast cancer was unchanged.

Overall, these results indicate that in women under the age of 50 extensive mammographic dysplasia is strongly associated with breast cancer, affects a substantial proportion of women with breast cancer, and this association is not modified by taking into account other risk factors for breast cancer.

The relationship of mammographic dysplasia to the histology of the mammary epithelium has been subjected to few systematic examinations. However, studies have shown an association (Wellings & Wolfe, 1978) between radiologic changes of dysplasia and histologic changes in mammary epithelium that are believed to be associated with an increased risk of breast cancer (Black, Barclay, Cutler, Hankey, & Asire, 1972; Wellings, Jensen & Marcun, 1975). This finding does not, of course, imply that the radiologic changes themselves represent changes in mammary epithelium, but only that the two are associated. However, this evidence does suggest that breast changes as seen on mammography might be employed as an indicator of risk that is at least potentially susceptible to change by dietary alteration, and might be useful as a target variable for testing hypotheses about the relationship between diet and breast cancer. Because of this evidence, we decided to examine one aspect of the relationship of dietary fat to mammary dysplasia, specifically to determine if a reduction in dietary fat maintained for one year could reduce the extensiveness of radiologic signs of mammary dysplasia. The specific objectives of our research were: (1) to assess the feasibility of recruiting women with breast dysplasia into a dietary program aimed at reducing dietary fat intake; (2) to assess compliance with the prescribed diet of those who entered the program; and (3) to assess the effect of reducing dietary fat intake on the clinical and radiologic features of breast dysplasia.

RESEARCH METHODS

Objective #1: Feasibility of Recruiting Women with Breast Dysplasia into a Dietary Program Aimed at Reducing Dietary Fat Intake. Women eligible for this study were identified in the Breast Diagnostic Unit and Surgical Wards of Women's College Hospital, Toronto, by the study research assistant with the consent of the patient's physician. Patients were eligible if they were aged over 30, had been judged to be free of breast cancer, had no personal history of breast cancer, and met the following criteria:

1. Had a mammogram in the previous three months that showed radiologic signs of mammary dysplasia occupying at least 50% of the breast volume.
2. The patient's physician planned to repeat clinical and mammographic examination in 12 months.

Patients who were on medically prescribed diets for any reason, or who were pregnant or breast feeding, were excluded, as were patients who habitually ate outside the home, or who lived outside Toronto.

The research assistant described the purposes of the study to eligible patients, and outlined the procedures to be employed. The purposes and methods of the study were described in a booklet that was left with the patient. We told the patients that we wished to study the effects of two types of diet on breast tissue, in the hope that this knowledge would provide information about how diet might be related to breast cancer. We explained that there was at present no evidence available to indicate that a dietary change could effect any alteration in benign breast disease. We did not say that various types of benign breast disease may confer an increased risk of breast cancer, and if they specifically asked about this, they were referred to their surgeon or family physician.

Patients were told that if they agreed to enter the study they would be selected to receive either general advice about their diet to ensure that they were eating a healthy diet as defined by government recommendations, or they would be selected to receive advice and teaching about buying and cooking foods in a way that reduced dietary fat intake, while at the same time preserving a healthy diet. Typical menus characterizing the type of low fat diet employed are shown in Table 10.3. It should however be stressed that these menus were used solely for the purposes of illustration and do not represent a diet that the patients were instructed to follow. As discussed further, we gave patients personal dietary instructions based upon individual food preferences, and told them that if either type of diet succeeded in bringing about a beneficial change in benign breast disease, and they were not allocated to receive that diet, they would be contacted at the end of the study and instructed in the successful diet.

Patients who agreed to enter the study after this explanation were randomly allocated to receive either the dietary assessment and general advice, or dietary

TABLE 10.3
Sample Menus for Diets

SAMPLE MENU - DIET I	SAMPLE MENU - DIET II
Breakfast	Breakfast
6 oz. orange juice 2 muffets 6 oz. skim milk 2 tsp. brown sugar coffee and skim milk and sugar	4 oz. orange juice 1 muffet 1 slice toast with jam 4 oz. whole milk 2 tsp. brown sugar 1 tsp. butter coffee and 10% cream and sugar
Lunch	Lunch
1 cup vegetable soup 2 slices of bread 2 tsp. butter 2 oz. lean cooked ham 1 apple coffee or tea with skim milk and sugar	½ cup cream of mushroom soup 2 slices bread 2 tsp. butter and one mayonnaise 2 oz. chicken salad 1 apple coffee and 10% cream and sugar
Dinner	Dinner
4 oz. of cooked chicken, fish, or lean meat 1 medium potato 1 dinner roll ½ cup cooked corn or peas 1 tsp. butter or margarine ½ cup green beans salad with fat free diet dressing ½ cup applesauce (sweetened) coffee or tea with skim milk and sugar	4 oz. of cooked meat 1 medium potato ½ cup of green beans salad with dressing butter on potatoes and beans ½ cup applesauce (sweetened) coffee or tea with milk and sugar
Evening Snack	Evening Snack
tea biscuit with jam - 1 tbsp. 6 oz. skim milk	crackers cheese whole milk

assessment and advice about reducing dietary fat consumption. At the time of randomization all patients entering the study were asked to provide information about their present diet, about demographic variables and risk factors for breast cancer, and about their history of previous breast symptoms and breast biopsies. The research assistant collected information about risk factors and other data at the time the patient entered the study. Dietary information was collected by the study dietitian whom patients visited at the Ludwig Institute.

Information about diet was collected in two ways, by a three day food record compiled by the patient, and by a diet history taken by the study dietitian using forms and methods developed by the Lipid Research Group. This information was recorded and coded by the study dietitians and the nutritional intake of each patient calculated by the Lipid Research Data Bank. The research assistant used a standard questionnaire to collect information about demographic variables, risk factors, and previous history of breast disease.

Additional procedures carried out at entry included breast examination, and recording the patient's weight, height, and triceps, subscapular, and iliac skin-fold thickness by the research assistant. Blood was taken by venipuncture for assays of cholesterol and storage for possible future assays of hormones.

The feasibility of recruiting women for the study was determined by comparing the number eligible and contacted by the research assistant with the number who sign the consent form to enter the study.

Objective #2: Assessment of Compliance with Prescribed Dietary Regimen. After entry into the study, patients were randomly assigned to one of two groups:

1. A group whose customary diet was assessed by the study dietitian, and advised of any adjustments required to make their diet conform to government recommendations concerning nutritional intake, and to achieve and maintain ideal body weight. This group of patients became the control group for the study.
2. A group of patients who were encouraged to reduce their dietary fat intake to the level where fat constituted 15% of total calories and to maintain this dietary change for 12 months. This group of patients formed the study or intervention group. The target level of 15% of calories as fat was selected because it is approximately the fat intake in countries where breast cancer incidence is lowest, and was judged to be the lowest level of fat intake consistent with a nutritionally balanced diet.

It is clear that to adequately test the effect of reduced dietary fat intake on mammary dysplasia, a substantial proportion of the patients in this group must achieve and maintain the prescribed dietary goals. The deployment of methods to promote compliance with these dietary goals was thus a crucial aspect of this study. The following specific measures, many of which have been developed and employed by the Lipid Research Group, were used:

1. The patient population selected was referred to Women's College Hospital with suspected breast disease and was expected to be receptive to the proposed trials.
2. The individual assessment of each patient's customary dietary pattern by the study dietitian allowed the personal development of proposed dietary changes

for patients, based upon individual dietary preferences, with personal instruction in the practical application of the diet.

3. Patients entering the intervention group were provided with written suggestions about shopping for low fat foods, recipes and menus suggesting a wide variety of meals, and suggestions about maintaining their diet while eating out.

4. Close contact was maintained on follow-up between the dietitian and each patient in the intervention group. Patients were given a phone number at which the dietitian or other study personnel could be contacted in case of difficulty, and were asked to visit the dietitian at the Institute two weeks after starting the diet, and then at intervals of one month for the duration of the study. At these visits the patients were asked to provide a three day food record. Their food intake over the previous 24 hours was reviewed, and encouragement, advice, and any necessary instruction provided. Compliance in the study group was assessed by determining the proportion of patients who, as judged by these repeated dietary assessments, consistently consumed 15% or less of calories as fat, and the proportions falling within each 5% increment from the target level. Particular attention was paid to the patients' weight on these visits and advice provided about ways of supplementing caloric intake without increasing fat consumption for any patients who fell below ideal body weight.

Patients in the control group were interviewed by the study dietitian at intervals of four months after entry, for a total of four assessments, including those at the beginning and end of the study. The purpose of these assessments was to determine if members of the control group had changed their dietary habits after entering the study.

Blood taken by venipuncture for measurement of serum cholesterol, and for storage for possible later hormone assays, was also obtained at monthly intervals in the intervention group and every 4 months in the control group. At the conclusion of 12 months patients in both intervention and control groups were asked to repeat a three day food record and to provide a dietary history to the study dietitian.

Objective #3: To Assess the Effect of Reducing Fat Intake on the Clinical and Radiologic Features of Breast Dysplasia. The principal method used to examine the influence of dietary fat reduction on mammary dysplasia will be the radiologic comparisons of mammograms from patients in the intervention and control groups taken at entry into the study and 12 months later. We plan to use two methods of comparing mammograms. In the first, the extent of radiologic dysplasia will be assessed independently by three radiologists and classified according to the proportion of the breast volume occupied by dysplastic change using radiologic films arranged in random sequence. The results of this classification will then be analyzed to determine if patients who received the low fat diet experienced any reduction in the extent of dysplasia over the course of 12 months, and to compare any reduction in the extent of dysplasia with that found in the control group.

In the second method of assessment, the radiologic films will be read in pairs (both films from each patient, taken at the beginning and end of the study), with reference to the time sequence in which they were taken, but without knowledge of whether the patients belonged to the dietary intervention or control group. Differences in the extent of dysplasia will then be analyzed with reference to the dietary group to which the patient belonged. In both methods of assessment dietary compliance will be taken into account in a subsidiary analysis.

Physical examination of the breast will be repeated by the patient's surgeon at the end of 12 months and the findings recorded and compared with those recorded at the time of entry. In addition, patients are asked to maintain a health diary recording menstrual history, and any illnesses experienced by the patient or her family during the course of the study.

Questions about the frequency, duration and severity of breast symptoms are repeated every four months throughout the study and compared with those at entry. The patient records these manifestations of breast disease in the health diary, which is maintained by both control and intervention groups and the severity of breast symptoms is also recorded using visual analog scales.

Sample Size

One hundred patients in each of the intervention and observation groups will allow the detection of a 25% reduction in dysplasia, with an alpha of 0.05 and a power of 0.95, assuming that not more than 5% of the observation group experienced such a reduction in dysplasia, and that compliance in the intervention group is at least 70%.

RESULTS

Only results bearing upon the feasibility of the study and compliance with the dietary intervention are presented. Analysis of the effects of dietary change upon mammographic and clinical manifestations of breast disease is presently being carried out.

Characteristics of the Population

The mean age of patients entering the study was 46.34 years. Of the 174 patients who have entered, 170 were white, and four were black. One hundred and two (59%) were married, 31 (18%) were never married, and 33 (19%) were separated or divorced. Five (3%) were widowed.

Feasibility

The study began in July 1980, and since then 285 eligible patients have been identified. Of these, 174 (61%) entered the study and consented to randomization. Seventy patients have completed a year on the study, and 61 patients, 9 from the control group and 22 from the intervention group, have dropped out. Of the patients who dropped out of the intervention group, 10 did so at the time of randomization and the remainder did so after being in the study for 3 to 5 months. Of the patients who dropped out of the control group, 3 did so at the time of randomization and the remainder at 4 months.

Fig.10.1 shows the mean total number of calories consumed as fat by the control and intervention groups over the course of the study to date. The number of patients whose data are shown is less than the total number enrolled because dietary information from the most recent patient visits is still being analyzed. In this and each of the following figures where mean values of nutrients are shown, the mean for each group is derived by first calculating a daily mean intake for each individual by averaging the calculated intake from the three day food record, and then pooling these values from individuals to generate a mean for the group as a whole.

At the time of randomization, the intervention group reported consuming a mean of 691 calories per day as fat (standard deviation 317 calories per day) and the control group a mean of 658 calories as fat (standard deviation 285 calories). Four months after randomization the intervention group reported an average intake of 328 calories a day as fat, a level that has been maintained with very little variation for the rest of the year. The mean fat intake of the control group

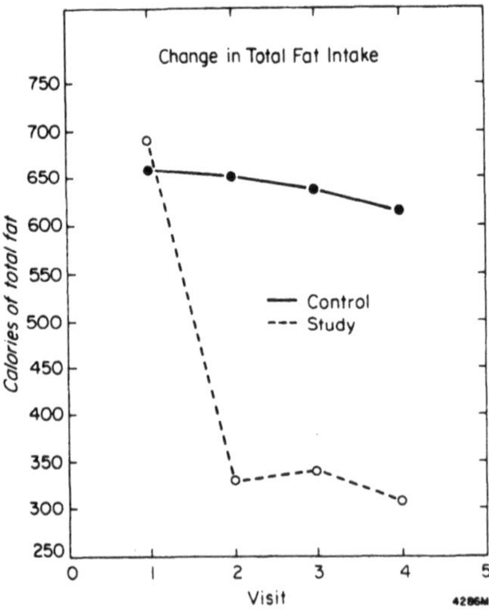

FIG. 10.1. Changes in mean fat intake in control and intervention groups.

has varied by no more than a few calories over the year, and differed significantly from the intervention group at each visit after the first ($p < 0.001$).

Fig. 10.2 shows the change in fat intake expressed as a percentage of total calories consumed as fat. At entry, both the intervention group and the control group reported consuming 37% of total calories as fat. The intake of the control group has remained relatively stable over the entire year of the study. By four months into the study, the intervention group had reduced their fat intake to a mean of 23% of calories, and this mean level has been maintained, or reduced slightly, over the course of a year and is significantly different ($p < 0.0001$) from the control.

Fig. 10.3 and 10.4 are histograms of fat intake, expressed as a percentage of total calories as fat, for the intervention and control groups. The frequencies shown are values for individual dietary records rather than for individual patients. Fig. 10.3 shows the distribution for the intervention and control groups at 0 and 4 months and Fig. 10.4 the data for months 8 and 12. At the time of randomization, intervention and control subjects showed a similar distribution of fat consumption with a mode around 37.5% of calories as fat. When assessed again four months after randomization the distribution of fat consumption of the intervention group showed a marked change, with a mode of 17.5% of calories as fat, and very few values at or above the initial modal level of 37.5. This general change in distribution has persisted through subsequent visits at 8 and 12 months. No change in the distribution of fat consumption has been observed in the control group.

Fig. 10.5 shows the total caloric intake of the study and control groups as assessed by the three day food record, compiled by each patient for each visit.

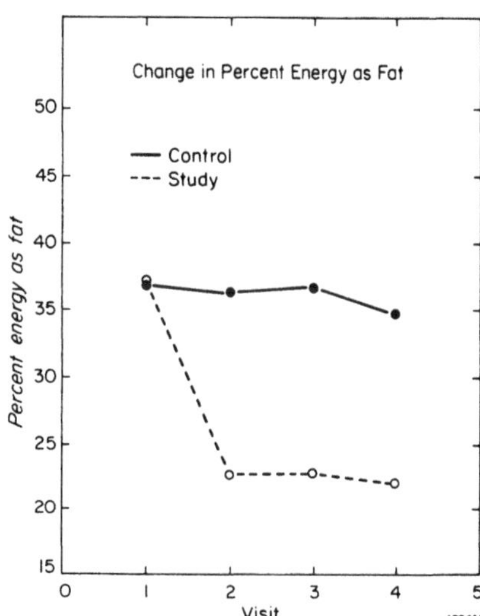

FIG. 10.2. Changes in mean energy intake as fat in control and intervention groups.

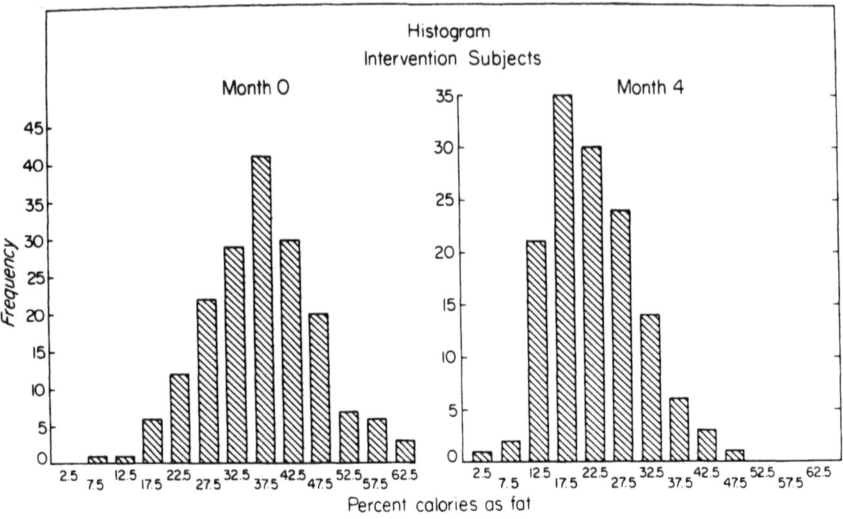

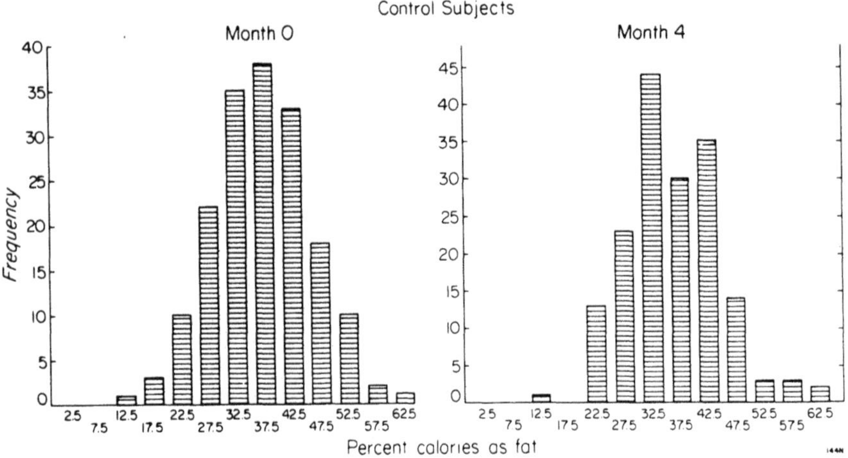

FIG. 10.3. Histogram of fat intake in intervention and control groups.

Caloric intake of the two groups was similar at the time of randomization and was similar to the caloric intake for Canadian women found in other studies (Beaton et al., 1979). After randomization the study group reported consuming about 250 calories per day less than the control group, a difference that is statistically significant ($p < 0.0001$).

Fig. 10.6 shows the mean values for serum cholesterol of the control and intervention groups. At entry, the mean serum cholesterol of the intervention group was slightly higher than that of the controls, but by four months had fallen

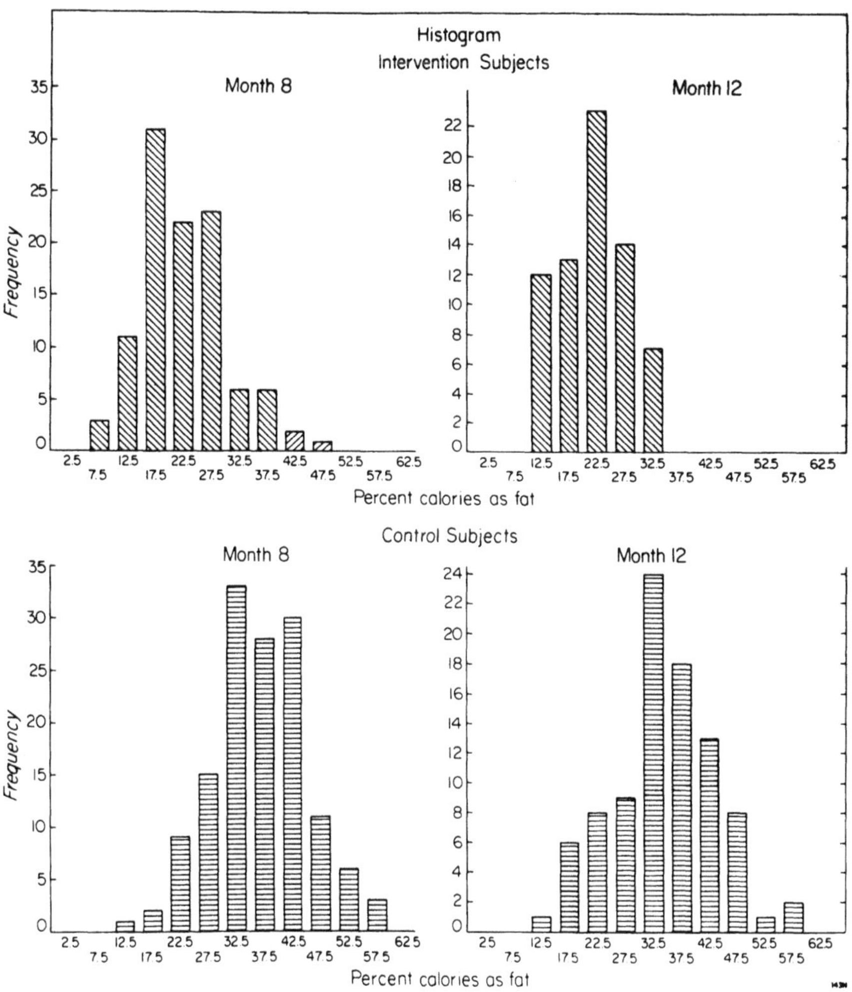

FIG. 10.4. Histogram of fat intake in control and intervention groups.

to about 20 mg below that of the controls, a difference that is statistically significant and has persisted for the remainder of the study.

Fig. 10.7 shows the mean weights of the control and intervention groups during the course of the study. Maintenance of weight is a concern, because substantial changes in weight might be accompanied by changes in breast size, which would give rise to difficulties when comparing mammograms taken at the beginning and the end of the study. However, weight is generally well maintained. The mean weight of the intervention group fell by 5 pounds over the course of a year, whereas that of the controls rose by 4 pounds.

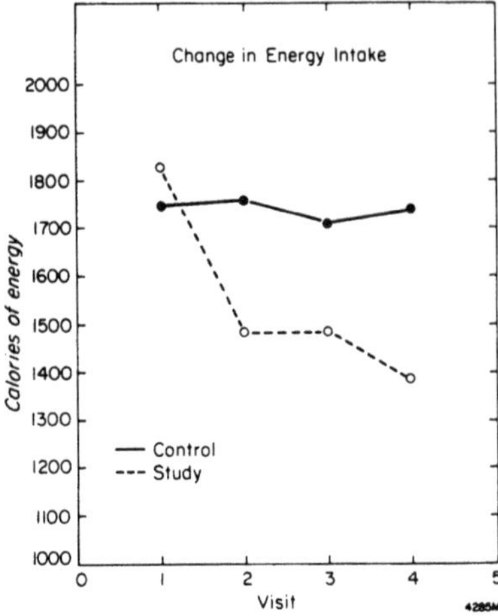

FIG. 10.5. Total caloric intake of intervention and control groups.

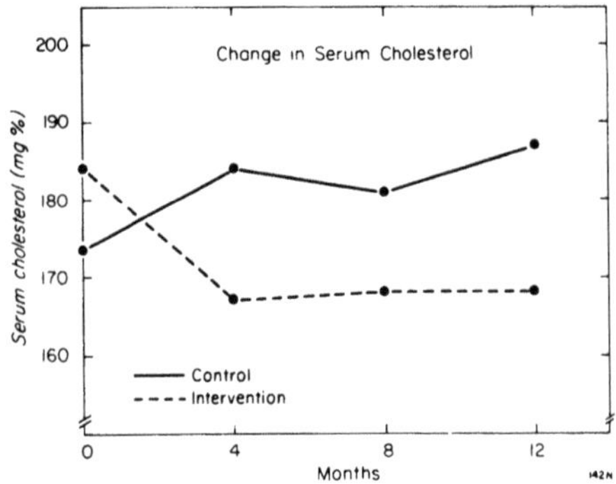

FIG. 10.6. Changes in mean serum cholesterol in control and intervention groups.

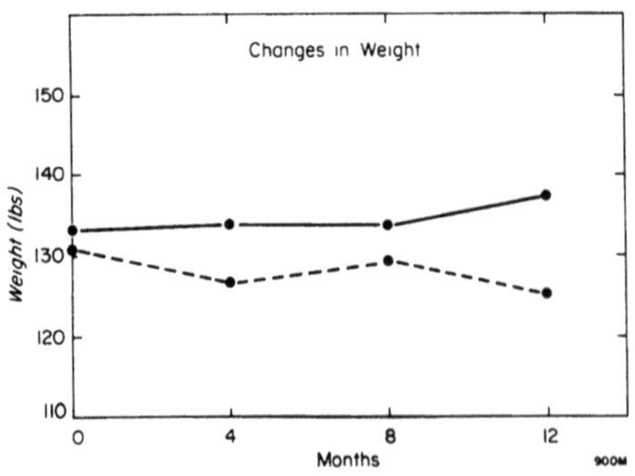

FIG. 10.7. Changes in body weight in control and intervention groups.

CONCLUSION

These results, although preliminary, indicate that it is feasible to attempt to study the effects of a major dietary intervention in a sizable free-living human population. The group of patients that we have chosen to study is unlikely to be typical of the general population, but is more likely to be interested in the possibility that a change in diet may help to relieve distressing symptoms of breast disease, even though we have avoided any suggestion that this is a likely outcome of the study. It also seems possible that patients may have been further motivated by accounts in the lay press describing the relationship between fat consumption and cancer risk. Nevertheless, it is unusual in any randomized clinical trial for such a high proportion of eligible subjects to consent to randomization.

Compliance with the dietary intervention, as assessed by food records and dietary recall, is close to the target set for the study, and although based upon patients' records, is corroborated by changes in serum cholesterol values. It thus appears that the methods used in this study to promote compliance are capable of effecting a substantial change in the diets of individuals. We are examining more closely the relationship between nutrient intake as assessed by food records and by more complex chemical measures including fecal fat, urinary methylhistidine (a measure of meat intake) (Jacobson, Newmark, Eyssen, & Bruce, 1983) and fasting serum lipids. All such measures, including food records, share the shortcoming that they provide estimates of nutrient intake only over a relatively brief period of time. However, as the maintenance of continuous food records over long periods of time is clearly impractical, the longterm assessment of diet will await the development of chemical measures that reflect longterm dietary practices.

It thus appears at this stage of the trial that well-motivated individuals can make a substantial and sustained alteration in their dietary habits, providing they are given sufficient support, advice, and education. It is likely that the close relationship established between patients and the study dietitians is an important element in achieving this level of compliance. Patients in the intervention group are asked to visit the dietitians monthly for a year and appear to find these visits useful sources of encouragement and advice. It is not at present clear whether such close supervision is necessary for longer term dietary interventions. Several patients who have completed a year in the intervention group report intolerance to dietary fat, and express an intention to maintain a reduced intake of dietary fat even though they are no longer in the study. We plan to reassess the diet of these individual's at intervals after the study has ended.

The effect, if any, of dietary change upon breast tissue cannot yet be assessed. However, an obvious and important gap in our present knowledge is the lack of any information about the relationship between change in radiologic appearances or clinical manifestations and changes in the histology of the breast epithelium. We are currently exploring the possibility of evaluating such changes by examining breast epithelial cells obtained by nipple aspiration and fine needle biopsy (Petrakis et al., 1981; Buehring, 1979). Several hypotheses about the role of diet in the etiology of cancer have been generated by epidemiologic and laboratory studies. The list of dietary factors suspected of contributing to the causation of cancer includes excesses of fat, protein and meat, and deficiencies of fiber, cruciferous vegetables, vitamins and selenium. To adequately test these several hypotheses as means of preventing cancer in human populations would be a formidable task requiring very large numbers of subjects followed over a long period of time. Studies of the type presented here, in which the reversal of a possible precursor lesion rather than the prevention of a malignant tumor is used as an endpoint, may offer a more feasible alternative.

REFERENCES

Armstrong, R. (1976). Recent trends in breast cancer incidence and mortality in relation to changes in possible risk factors. *International Journal of Cancer, 17,* 204–211.

Armstrong, B., & Doll, R. (1975). Environmental factors and cancer incidence and mortality in different countries with special reference to dietary practices. *International Journal of Cancer, 15,* 617–631.

Bailar, J. C. III (1977). Screening for early breast cancer: Pros and cons. *Cancer, 39,* 2783–2795.

Beaton, G. H., Milner, J., Corey, P., McGuire, V., Cousins, M., Stewart, E., de Ramos, M., Hewitt, D., Grambsch, P. V., Kassim, N., & Little, J. A. (1979). Sources of variance in 24 hour dietary recall data: Implications for nutrition study design and interpretation. *American Journal of Clinical Nutrition, 31* (12), 2456–2559.

Bjarnason, O., Day, N., & Snaedal, G., & Tulinius, H. (1974). The effect of year of birth on the breast cancer age-incidence curve in Iceland. *International Journal of Cancer, 13,* 689–696.

Black, M. M., Barclay, T. H. C., Cutler, S. J., Hankey, B. F., & Asire, A. J. (1972). Association of atypical characteristics of benign breast lesions with frequent risk of breast cancer. *Cancer, 29,* 338–343.

Boyd, N. F., O'Sullivan, B., Campbell, J. E., Fishell, E., Simor, I., Cooke, G., & Germanson, T. (1982a). Bias and the association of mammographic parenchymal patterns with breast cancer. *British Journal of Cancer, 45,* 179–184.

Boyd, N. F., O'Sullivan, B., Campbell, J. E., Fishell, E., Simor, I., Cooke, G., & Germanson, T. (1982b). Mammographic signs as risk factors for breast cancer. *British Journal of Cancer, 45,* 185–193.

Boyd, N. F., O'Sullivan, B., Campbell, J. E., Fishell, E., Simor, I., Cooke, G., & Germanson, T. (1982c) Mammographic patterns and bias in breast cancer detection. *Radiology, 143*(3), 671–674.

Boyd, N.F., O'Sullivan, B., Fishell, E., Simor, I., & Cooke, G. (1984). Mammographic patterns and breast cancer risk: Methodologic standards and contradictory results. *Journal of the National Cancer Institute, 72*(6), 1253–1259.

Brisson, J., Sadowsky, N. L., Twaddle, J. A., Morrison, A. S., Cole, P., & Merletti, F. (1982). Mammographic features of the breast and breast cancer risk. *American Journal of Epidemiology, 115,* 428–437.

Bruce, W. R., Eyssen, G. M., Ciampi, A., Dion, D. W., & Boyd, N.F. (1981) Strategies for dietary intervention studies in colon cancer. *Cancer, 47,* 1121–1125.

Buehring, G. C. (1979). Screening for breast atypias using exfoliative cytology. *Cancer, 43,* 1788–1799.

Buell, P. (1973). Changing incidence of breast cancer in Japanese-American women. *Journal of the National Cancer Institute, 51,* 1479–1483.

Carroll, K. K., Gammell, E. B., & Plunkett, E. R. (1968). Dietary fat and mammary cancer. *Canadian Medical Association Journal, 98,* 590–594.

Carroll, K. K., & Khor, H. T. (1975). Dietary fat in relation to tumorigenesis. *Progress and Biochemical and Pharmacology, 10,* 308–353.

Chaudary, M. A., Gravelle, I. H., Bulstrode, J. C., Wang, D. Y., Millis, R. R., & Hayward, J. L. (1983). Breast parenchymal patterns in women with bilateral primary breast cancer. *British Journal of Radiology, 56,* 703–706.

Devesa, S. A. & Silverman, D. T. (1978). Cancer incidence and mortality trends in the United States 1935–74. *Journal of the National Cancer Institute, 60,* 545–571.

Doll, R., Muir, C., & Waterhouse, J. (Eds.), (1976). *Cancer incidence in five continents.* IARC Scientific Publication.

Doll, R., & Peto, R. (1981). The causes of cancer: Quantitative estimates of avoidable risks of cancer in the United States today. *Journal of the National Cancer Institute, 66,* 1193–1265.

Drasar, B. S., & Irving, D. (1973). Environmental factors and cancer of the colon and breast. *British Journal of Cancer, 27,* 167–172.

Ernster, V. I., Sack, S. T., Peterson, C. A. & Schweitzer, R. J., (1980). Mammographic parenchymal patterns and risk factors for breast cancer. *Radiology, 134,* 617–620.

Fisher, B., Redmond, C. Brown, A., Wolmark, N., Wittliff, J., Fisher, E. R., Plotkin, D., Bowman, D., Sachs, S., Wolter, J., Frelich, R., Desser, R., LiCalzi, N., Geggie, P. Campbell, T., Elias, E. G., Prager, D., Koontz, P., Volk, H., Kimitrov, N., Gardner, B., Lerner, H., & Shibata, H. (1981). Treatment of primary breast cancer with chemotherapy and Tamoxifen. *New England Journal of Medicine, 305,* 1–6.

Graham, S., Marshall, J., & Mettlin, C. (1982). Diet in the epidemiology of breast cancer. *American Journal of Epidemiology, 116,* 68–75.

Gray, G. E., Pike, M. C., & Henderson, B. E. (1981). Dietary fat and plasma prolactin. *American Journal of Clinical Nutrition, 34,* 1160–1162.

Haenszel, W., & Kurihara, M. (1968). Studies of Japanese migrants. I. Mortality from cancer and other diseases among Japanese in the United States. *Journal of the National Cancer Institute, 40,* 43–68.

Hainline, S., Myers, L., McLelland, R., Newell, J., Grufferman, S., & Shingleton, W. (1978). Mammographic patterns and risk of breast cancer. *American Journal of Roentgenology, 130,* 1157–1158.

Hill, P., & Wynder, E. L. (1976). Diet and prolactin release. *Lancet, 2,* 806–807.

Hirayama, T. (1979). Diet and cancer. *Nutrition and Cancer, 1*(3), 67–81.

Hopkins, G. J., & West, C. E. (1976). Possible roles of dietary fats in carcinogenesis. *Life Sciences, 19*(8), 1103–1116.

Jacobson, E. A., Newmark, H. L., Eyssen, G. H., & Bruce, W. R. (1983). Estimation of 3-Methylhistidine in urine as an estimate of meat consumption. *Nutritional Reports International, 27,* 689–697.

Kelsey, J. L. (1979). A review of the epidemiology of human breast cancer. In P. E. Sartwell (Ed.), *Epidemiologic reviews, 1* (pp. 74–109). Baltimore: Johns Hopkins University Press.

Krook, P. M. (1975). Mammographic parenchymal patterns as risk indicators for incident cancer in a screening program: An extended analysis. *American Journal of Radiology, 131,* 1031–1035.

Krook, P. M., Carlile, T., Bush, W., & Hall, M. H. (1978). Mammographic parenchymal patterns as a risk indicator for prevalent and incident cancer. *Cancer, 41,* 1093–1097.

Lea, A. J. (1966). Dietary factors associated with death rates from certain neoplasms in man. *Lancet, 2,* 332–333.

Mendell, L., Rosenbloom, M., & Naimark, A. (1977). Are breast patterns a risk index for breast cancer? A reappraisal. *American Journal of Roentgenology, 128,* 547.

Miller, A. B. (1977). Role of nutrition in the etiology of breast cancer. *Cancer, 39,* 2704–2708.

Miller, A. B., Kelly, A., Choi, N. W., Matthers, V., Morgan, R. W., Munan, L., Burch, J. D., Feather, J., Howe, G. R., & Jain, M. (1978). A study of diet and breast cancer. *American Journal of Epidemiology, 107,* 499–509.

Miller, A. B., Howe, G. R., Wall, C. (1981). The national study of breast screening. Protocol for a Canadian randomized controlled trial of screening for breast cancer in women. *Clinical and Investigative Medicine, 4,* 227–258.

Moskowitz, M., Gartside, P., & McLaughlin, C. (1980). Mammographic patterns as markers for high-risk benign breast disease and incident cancer. *Radiology, 134,* 293-295.

Mueller, C. B., & Jeffries, W. (1975). Cancer of the breast: Its outcome as measured by rate of dying and cause of death. *Annals of Surgery, 182,* 334–341.

Mukai, F. M. & Goldstein, B. D. (1976). Mutagenicity of Malonaldehyde, a decomposition product of peroxidized polyunsaturated fatty acids. *Sciences, 191,* 868–869.

Petrakis, N. L., Ernster, V. L. Sacks, S. T., King, E. B., Schweitzer, R. J., Hunt, T. K., & King, M. C. (1981). Epidemiology of breast fluid secretion: Association with breast cancer risk factors and cerumen type. *Journal of the National Cancer Institute, 67,* 277–284.

Phillips, R. L. (1975). Role of life style and dietary habits in risk of cancer among Seventh-Day Adventists. *Cancer Research, 35,* 3513–3522.

Pike, M. C., Siiteri, P. K., & Welsch, C. W. (Eds.) (1981). *Hormones and breast cancer.* Banbury Report 8. Cold Spring Harbor Laboratory.

Reddy, B. S., Cohen, L. A., McCoy, G. D., Hill, P. M., Weisburger, J. H., & Wynder, E. L. (1980). *Nutrition and its relationship to cancer. Advances in cancer research.* In: G Klein (Ed.), (Volume 32). New York: Academic Press.

Rideout, D. F. & Poon, P. Y. (1977). Patterns of breast parenchyma on mammography. *Journal Canadian Association of Radiology, 28,* 257–258.

Rossi, A., Bonnadonna, G., Valagussa, P., & Veronesi, V. (1981). Multimodal treatment in operable breast cancer: 5 year result of the CMF programme. *British Medical Journal, 282,* 1427–1431.

Shapiro, S. (1977). Evidence of screenings for breast cancer from a randomized trial. *Cancer, 39,* 2772–2782.

Tannenbaum, A. (1942) The genesis and growth of tumours IV. Effects of a high fat diet. *Cancer Research, 2,* 468–475.

Tannenbaum, A., & Silverstone H. (1957). In R. W. Raven (Ed.), *Cancer,* Vol. 1 (pp. 306–334).

Threatt, B., Norbeck, J. M., Ullman, N. S., Kummer, R., & Rosell, P. (1980). Assocation between mammographic parenchymal pattern classification and incidence of breast cancer. *Cancer, 45,* 2550–2556.

Toppler, Y. J., & Freeman, C. S. (1980). Multiple hormone interactions in the developmental biology of the mammary gland. *Physiological Reviews, 69,* 1049–1106.

Urbanski, S., Cooke, G., Jensen, H. M., McFarlane, D., Wellings, S. R., & Boyd, N. F. (In preparation). *Histologic and radiologic indicators of breast cancer risk.*

Wellings, S. R., & Wolfe, J. N. (1978). Correlation studies of the histological and radiographic appearances of the breast parenchyma. *Radiology, 129,* 299–306.

Wellings, S. R., Jensen, H. M., & Marcum, R. G. (1975). An atlas of syndrome pathology of the human breast with special preference to the possible precancerous lesions. *Journal of the National Cancer Institute, 55,* 231–273.

Wilkinson, E., Clopton, C., Gordonson, J., Green, R., Hill, A., & Pike, M. C. (1977). Mammographic parenchymal pattern and the risk of breast cancer. *Journal of the National Cancer Institute, 59,* 1397–1400.

Williams, R. H., (Ed.) (1968). *Textbook of endocrinology.* Philadelphia: Saunders.

Wolfe, J. N. (1976). Breast patterns as an index of risk for developing breast cancer. *American Journal of Roentgenology, 126,* 1130–1139.

Wolfe, J. N., Albert, S., Belle, S., & Salane, M. (1982). Breast parenchymal patterns: Analysis of 332 incident breast carcinomas. *American Journal or Roentgenology, 138,* 113–118.

11 The Influence of Nutritional Intervention on the Outcome of Cancer Treatment

Arthur S. Levine, M.D.
National Institutes of Health

INTRODUCTION

Nutrition and cancer have a number of intersections. With regard to etiology and pathogenesis, it is increasingly evident that there is a relationship between our intake of certain foodstuffs and the development of various types of cancer. For example, in certain high risk countries, a link has been demonstrated between the increased intake of fat (with a decrease in fiber content) and the development of colon cancer (Rivlin, Shils, & Sherlock, 1983). Increased fat intake has also been associated with the development of breast cancer, and in experimental animals as well as epidemiologically, there is evidence that the absence of certain trace elements and vitamins may correlate with the occurrence of various cancers (Rivlin et al., 1983).

At another level, patients with cancer may develop secondary abnormalities that affect their nutrition. For example, the presence of cancer per se, or even the fear of the presence of cancer, may induce psychological reactions that might alter the dietary intake adversely. Patients with head and neck cancer may not be able to swallow, and those with cancer of the gastrointestinal tract may develop an obstruction to the passage of food or malabsorption of the nutrients (Costa & Donaldson, 1979). Importantly, some patients with cancer experience significant but poorly understood metabolic changes which compromise their nutritional status; we may find weight loss and malnutrition as well as deficiencies of individual nutrients in such patients (Brennan, 1981, 1982). Indeed, the mechanism of cachexia and "the catabolic state" in cancer patients remain major unsolved problems. A description of the localized and systemic affects of neoplastic diseases on nutritional status is presented in Table 11.1. In reviewing this

TABLE 11.1

Some Effects of Neoplastic Diseases on Nutritional Status

Malnutrition secondary to persistent anorexia.
Malnutrition associated with impaired food intake secondary to obstruction.
Malabsorption associated with:
  Deficiency of pancreatic enzymes or bile salts.
  Infiltration of small bowel by neoplasms, such as lymphoma or carcinoma.
  Fistulous bypass of small bowel.
Protein-losing enteropathy (in gastric carcinoma or lymphoma or with lymphatic obstruction).
Electrolyte and fluid balance disturbances associated with:
    Persistent vomiting in obstruction.
    Vomiting secondary to increased intracranial pressure from tumors.
    Small bowel fluid losses from fistula.
    Diarrhea associated with hormone-secreting tumors and villous adenoma of the colon.

Modified from Rivlin et al. (1983).

list, note that the high incidence and prolonged, deleterious effects of anorexia are of particular significance. Although the causes of anorexia remain uncertain, it is possible that peptides known to affect appetite are secreted in tumor-bearing hosts (Rivlin et al., 1983). The metabolic changes in neoplastic disease may, in addition to depressing food intake, alter energy metabolism (Brennan, 1981, 1982; Copeland, Daly, Ota, & Dudrick, 1979; Costa & Donaldson, 1979; Rivlin et al., 1983; Steiger, Oram-Smith, Miller, Kuo, & Vars, 1975; Hays, Merritt, White, Ashley, & Siegel, 1983). Requirements are increased beyond those of normal persons of otherwise similar status. Thus, cancer patients may behave like patients who are hypercatabolic for other reasons, exhibiting decreased protein synthesis and negative nitrogen balance with the food intake that would sustain a normal person (Brennan, 1982). A durable and total reversal of the undesirable nutritional changes secondary to the effects of cancer is dependent upon regression or cure of the underlying malignant disease. There is no question, however, that these effects can be mitigated in a number of simple ways, such as the use of ethnic foods, the serving of larger portions at times remote from chemotherapy-induced nausea, and the use of nutritional supplements. More complex and sophisticated procedures, such as enteral feeding (by oral tube) and total parenteral nutrition (i.e., the total requirement of nutrients delivered intravenously) also have much to offer in the appropriate circumstances.

These maneuvers may decrease morbidity and shorten convalescence (Brennan, 1981, 1982; Copeland et al., 1979; Costa & Donaldson, 1979; Hays, Merritt, White, Ashley, & Siegel, 1983).

Significant nutritional problems may also arise as the result of the specific mode of treatment given to control the cancer (Brennan, 1982; Costa & Donaldson, 1979; Rivlin et al., 1983). For example, radiation to the head and neck may destroy the sense of taste, and radiation to the bowel may produce malabsorption and obstruction. Surgical removal of portions of the gastrointestinal tract may produce malabsorption, diarrhea, or swallowing difficulties. Cancer chemotherapeutic agents commonly produce anorexia, nausea, vomiting, damaged mucosal surfaces and ulcers, as well as diarrhea. The degree to which chemotherapeutic agents adversely affect intestinal functions depends on the dosage, the frequency and duration of treatment, the rates of metabolism, and the specific drugs involved. Most chemotherapeutic regimens are prolonged for several years and therefore the impairment in food intake may be chronic. The effects of such regimens are compounded by the use of chemotherapeutic agents in multi-combinations, delivered in high doses in a cyclic fashion. However, this method of administration appears to be the optimum form of chemotherapy in a number of malignant diseases, and has produced great improvements in disease-free and overall survival (Costa & Donaldson, 1979). The undesirable reactions to chemotherapy are more intense in patients with radiation effects on intestinal integrity or surgical removal of a portion of the intestinal tract.

Whether compromised nutrition is due to cancer and/or its treatment, even patients with less than an optimal response to nutritional support appear to do better in terms of weight and strength than those to whom no nutritional support is provided. This is particularly true for patients who are already significantly malnourished prior to cancer therapy. However, a more far-reaching question in studies of nutritional intervention in cancer patients is whether such intervention will prolong life significantly. Controlled clinical trials of total parenteral nutrition (TPN) may serve as a paradigm in addressing this question (Brennan, 1981).

It is evident that certain basic assumptions underlie treatment regimens which employ TPN in an attempt to improve the response to cancer therapy (Brennan, 1982). The first assumption is that the tumor and/or its therapy, whether surgery, chemotherapy, or radiotherapy, induces some degree of malnutrition. A second assumption is that the malnutrition is reversible by a manipulation such as TPN. The most important assumption is that if nutritional defects are corrected, tolerance to cancer therapy will improve, i.e., either the dose or dose rate (or both) of the cancer treatment can be increased.

Most cancer treatment regimens compromise the number and function of normal bone marrow cells. The tolerance of normal marrow, as well as other normal tissues, determines the intensity of chemotherapy that may be employed in each patient. Nutritional intervention during cancer treatment might improve the tolerance of bone marrow cells and other normal tissues to cancer treatment, and therefore permit a higher peak dose and/or cumulative dose. In the case of malignant diseases that demonstrate a linear dose–response curve, this approach might yield, in any population of cancer patients, a higher complete remission rate and/or longer relapse-free survival. In essence, these assumptions reflect the notion that there are at least some tumors, at some point in their natural histories, that demonstrate a relatively linear dose–response relationship. A major reason for failing to achieve effective tumoricidal doses or dose rates on this linear plot would be failure to correct a nutritional deficiency (Copeland et al., 1979). It is this notion which trials of nutritional intervention (or of any supportive care maneuver) in cancer patients must address directly (Levine & Deisseroth, 1978; Pizzo & Levine, 1977). However, it must be noted that in some studies involving animal tumor models, a change in nutritional status has favored the tumor rather than the host (Steiger et al., 1975). In this regard, Goldie and Coldman (1979) have proposed that drug resistance may relate to the spontaneous rate of somatic mutation within tumor cells. If an improvement in nutrition were to enhance the proliferative rate of the tumor, this increased rate might reflect an increase in the rate at which somatic mutation occurs, favoring drug resistance.

TOTAL PARENTERAL NUTRITION

TPN is widely used in situations in which nutritional support is not possible by the enteral route. Many claims have been made regarding the ability of TPN to reverse malnutrition in a vast number of disease states (Brennan, 1981, 1982). TPN can be performed safely, effectively, and with considerable nutritional benefit. However, as noted previously, the readily accepted nutritional benefits of TPN to the patient may not necessarily mean that TPN contributes meaningfully to the long-term outcome of the disease with which the malnutrition is associated.

Standard TPN mixtures include Freamine (amino acids), dextrose, electrolytes, calcium gluconate, iron dextran, vitamin B complex, vitamin C, trace metals, magnesium sulfate, folic acid, and insulin. Essential fatty acid deficiency will occur unless supplementation with an intravenous lipid solution is also provided (Brennan, 1982). Conventionally, the TPN mixture is administered via the subclavian vein.

The pioneering efforts of Copeland et al. (1979) did much to emphasize the efficacy and safety of TPN in the cancer patient. Moreover, in their earliest studies, they identified a benificial effect on response to chemotherapy in lung cancer patients who had a prior weight loss exceeding 6% of pre-illness body weight. Historical results were used as a basis for comparison. In another study, patients with greater than 10 pounds of weight loss prior to surgery for gastrointestinal malignancy were randomly assigned to receive either conventional nutritional support or TPN. These authors showed no difference in mortality or in complications whether the patient was in the TPN group or the control group (reviewed in Brennan, 1982). They were, however, able to demonstrate improvement in conventional indices of nutrition, such as serum albumin, and to lessen postoperative weight loss. A similar study examined the use of TPN in preoperative management of patients with gastric cancer. The mortality in the control group was 23%, whereas in the TPN treated group it was 14%. In addition, the incidence of wound infection in the TPN group was 6%, and in the control population, 26% (Reviewed in Costa & Donaldson, 1979). This is one of the few controlled studies in the literature to suggest that nutritional support may be of value in the outcome of therapy for malignancy. Other studies examining the use of TPN as an adjunct to chemotherapy have shown that therapy-induced bone marrow suppression is significantly less in patients receiving TPN, but survival is not improved (Brennan, 1981, 1982; Copeland et al., 1979; Costa & Donaldson, 1979). These studies were, in general, not concurrently controlled. In a pediatric trial, immunological function, as assessed by skin test reactivity, total and "T" lymphocyte populations, and the mitogenic response to phytohemagglutinin, was believed to be improved by TPN (Hays et al., 1983).

On the other hand, a number of reports have noted the failure of nutritional support to influence in any way the course of cancer treatment (Brennan, 1981, 1982; Rivlin et al., 1983). For example, Copeland et al., in a second retrospectively controlled study of adults with radiation-treated lung cancer, found no improvement in tumor response nor in survival as a function of adjuvant TPN (Copeland et al., 1979). In a study of children with various tumors, no benefit from TPN was apparent with respect to tolerance to chemotherapy (Hays et al., 1983). Very few of these "negative" studies employed randomly assigned concurrent control patients, but most utilized retrospective comparisons, as had the "positive" trials. In other studies, patients were allowed to develop nutritional depletion prior to nutritional intervention, confounding an interpretation of the outcome of nutritional intervention.

It has only been in the past few years that prospectively randomized studies of TPN as an adjunct to cancer treatment have been undertaken, and the definitive results of such studies are now being reported. Because the impact of TPN on ultimate survival may not be large, and because of the number of potentially confounding variables in the complex clinical setting of cancer and its therapy, it is probable that the value of TPN or other nutritional interventions will only be demonstrated or refuted unequivocally in randomized studies. Thus, earlier clinical research in this area, while very helpful in the development of the relevant technology, has been limited in the inferences that these studies permit us to reach.

Meaningful clinical trials of nutritional intervention in cancer patients require that the tumor be responsive (i.e., at the maximum achievable dose and/or dose rate, a significant number of tumor regressions must ensue). Moreover, this dose or dose rate must not be achievable unless nutritional defects are corrected. In essence, the responsive tumor is not permitted to respond mainly because of the nutritional status of the host (Costa & Donaldson, 1979). It is evident that controlled clinical trials of TPN in cancer patients must therefore be stratified with respect to the type of tumor being studied, since tumors are differentially responsive to various treatments, and different tumors may be differentially associated with malnutrition. Tumor stage (the extent of spread) and other known prognostic variables must also be stratified. Ideally, such trials should involve one potentially responsive tumor at one point in its natural history, with all patients comparably staged and otherwise comparable for known prognostic variables. Other known variables which affect treatment tolerance, response, and survival, e.g., infection, antecedent weight loss, and gastrointestinal toxicity must also be stratified. Finally, one must consider the effect of other supportive care modalities, such as antibiotics, isolation rooms (designed to reduce the incidence of infectious complications), bone marrow transplantation, and white blood cell transfusion (Levine & Deisseroth, 1978; Pizzo & Levine, 1977); each one of these supportive care modalities, because it may improve the tolerance to therapy in any given patient, competes with TPN and therefore potentially clouds our understanding of the utility of TPN. Finally, there are assuredly unknown prognostic variables as well as those that can be identified. Since the impact of TPN on ultimate survival may be modest, it is evident that this modest effect will be demonstrated unequivocally only in prospectively randomized studies. Patients in both groups of such studies would be treated identically except for the one variable of nutritional intervention; both groups would be treated very intensively. Dose and/or dose rate would be escalated only in those patients who had tolerated the lower dose and/or dose rate.

In an attempt to meet these criteria for an appropriate study design, two prospectively randomized clinical trials have been initiated at the National Cancer Institute to assess the role of TPN in cancer treatment. Impetus for these studies was provided by the data in Tables 11.2 and 11.3 indicating an average weight loss of 18% prior to TPN in 80 unselected NCI patients and a mean daily pre-TPN intake in 34 unselected NCI patients of only 1587 total non-protein calories (i.e., the weight loss is predominantly due to diminished intake). In the design of both trials, the investigators sought to determine whether patients were

TABLE 11.2
Average Weight Loss Pre-TPN in 80 Unselected NCI Patients

Preillness weight	66.0 ± 1.8 kg
Pre-TPN weight	53.3 ± 2.0 kg
Weight loss	11.9 ± 1.2 kg
Average weight loss	18%

From Brennan (1982).

TABLE 11.3
Mean Daily Pre-TPN Intake in 34 Unselected NCI Patients

	IV	*Oral*	*Total*
Carbohydrate (gm)	128	215	343
Protein (gm)	---	51	51
Fat (gm)	---	35	35
Total nonprotein calories	436	1151	1587

From Brennan (1982).

initially debilitated, whether the debilitation was reversible with TPN, and whether (in the presence or absence of debilitation) TPN permitted an increased chemotherapy dose or dose rate—which in turn might yield an improved durable survival. TPN was employed in both studies (as opposed to other forms of adjunctive nutritional support) because all patients were to be treated with aggressive combination chemotherapy regimens that produce intense and protracted nausea and vomiting, precluding optimal oral supplementation. While the two NCI trials are prospectively randomized, other factors have still interfered with the drawing of definitive conclusions. A detailed discussion of these trials thus will illustrate the complexities and frustrations inherent in this area of clinical research.

NCI TRIAL OF TPN IN ADVANCED STAGES OF DIFFUSE LYMPHOMAS

The first prospectively randomized clinical trial of TPN undertaken at the NCI (1977) involved adult patients with advanced stages of diffuse, aggressive lymphomas other than Hodgkin's disease (Popp, Fisher, Simon, & Brennan, 1981; Popp, Fisher, Wesley, & Brennan, 1981). Non-Hodgkin's lymphomas (NHL) are among the human tumors which are most responsive to chemotherapy. Yet until recently, about half of all lymphoma patients did not experience a complete clinical remission and had a quick recurrence of their disease; the duration of their survival was consequently short. Even those patients who did experience a complete clinical remission sometimes had clinically undetectable tumor cells remaining at the microscopic level. Frequently these patients also had tumor recurrence and a relatively short survival. Thus, it has been widely held that NHL, although relatively responsive to chemotherapy, must still be treated more intensively if there is to be a further significant gain in survival. In 1977, these lymphomas appeared to be a good model for studies of nutritional intervention because although they were relatively responsive to chemotherapy, there was room for improvement.

In earlier studies, NHL patients treated initially at the NCI with five-drug regimens experienced a 46% complete tumor remission rate; 38% survived free of disease and off therapy at 5 years (Fisher, DeVita, Johnson, Simon, & Young, 1977). Since 1977, patients with advanced stages of diffuse NHL have been treated in the Medicine Branch of the NCI with the "ProMACE-MOPP" chemotherapy regimen (Fisher, DeVita, Hubbard, Brennan, Chabner, Simon, & Young, 1980) (see [1]for a definition of the acronym). This study was designed to increase the complete remission rates and, therefore, the long-term survival of patients with aggressive lymphomas by treatment with ProMACE induction therapy (consisting of a new regimen of active drugs), MOPP consolidation therapy with a known effective regimen which does not contain any of the drugs used in the induction regimen, and aggressive late intensification with the initial ProMACE induction regimen. The ProMACE regimen consists of five agents, administered cyclically with each cycle lasting 28 days. The five drugs have different mechanisms of action, presenting multiple opportunities for tumor cell killing but different types of side-effects. Rest periods between cycles permit recovery from the side-effects of these potent chemotherapeutic agents, especially recovery of the bone marrow's capacity to produce white and red blood cells and platelets. Not all patients respond to chemotherapy at the same rate, so the duration of the patient's induction, consolidation, or late intensification therapy with ProMACE-MOPP was tailored to the responsiveness of the patient's particular tumor. Patients who achieved a clinical remission slowly would receive more therapy than those whose rate of response was more rapid. A patient would remain on a given phase of this therapy until the rate of response of his or her tumor decreased or complete remission was achieved. In addition, patients entering the ProMACE-MOPP trial were randomized to receive either total parenteral nutrition or a standard diet in order to determine the role of hyperalimentation (intensive nutritional support) in preventing weight loss, improving nutritional status, permitting increased chemotherapy dosage, and increasing the complete response rate and long-term survival of these patients.

As in earlier NCI trials in the diffuse lymphomas, the majority of patients in this trial (70%) had diffuse histiocytic lymphoma, and about 60% had widely disseminated tumor masses. Analysis of the results of the ProMACE-MOPP regimen now indicates that the pathologically documented complete response rate has increased from 46% to 72%, with the complete response rate higher in each prognostic category. Moreover, actuarial analyses predict an increase in the number of patients cured of their disease from 38% to approximately 60% (Fisher et al., 1980; Popp, Fisher, Wesley, & Brennan, 1981).

Of 42 patients with advanced diffuse lymphoma, 21 were randomly selected to receive adjuvant TPN during the ProMACE-MOPP study. Fifty-six TPN

[1]The abbreviations used are: TPN, total parenteral nutrition; NCI, National Cancer Institute; MOPP, nitrogen mustard-vincristine-procarbazine-prednisone; ProMACE, prednisone-methotrexate-Adriamycin-cyclophosphamide-VP-16; DTIC, dimethyl-triazeno imidazole carboxamide.

courses were given during the first 14 days of the 28-day ProMACE induction and late-intensification cycles. The other 21 patients received conventional oral nutrition. About 20% of the members of each group had a prior weight loss exceeding 6% of pre-illness body weight, and thus could be defined as mildly malnourished at the inception of the study. Because of significant bone marrow suppression, all patients required dose modifications during treatment. One aim of the study was to determine whether patients receiving TPN would be able to tolerate a greater drug dosage and if, as a consequence, the overall tumor response would be enhanced.

TPN patients received an average of 2200 kcal/day and ate an additional 800 kcal/day during therapy. These patients had marked weight gains, whereas conventional-diet patients had stable weights both during induction and late intensification cycles and over the entire course of therapy. Lean body mass, as indicated by total body potassium, anthropomorphic measurements, and other assays, was not improved in TPN patients as compared to control patients. These results suggest that the weight gained by TPN patients was composed of fat, water or both. Although TPN might protect against treatment-induced bone marrow suppression and in this way improve the tolerance to marrow-suppressive chemotherapy, the median nadir of the white blood cell count, and the time taken to achieve this nadir, were not different between the two study groups. Thus, in this trial, TPN did not promote marrow recovery and on this basis would not have permitted more intensive treatment.

The dose of the chemotherapeutic agents to be administered was decreased only according to predetermined toxicity guidelines. Thus, a comparison of drug dosage in the group receiving TPN and the group receiving conventional oral nutrition is a measure of drug tolerance in these patients. In fact, no difference in tolerance of any specific drug or total drug dose occurred when all patients in both groups were compared. Similar comparisons in subgroups of malnourished patients and responding patients also revealed no difference. Moreover, a cycle-by-cycle analysis demonstrated no difference in any phase of therapy. As a group, TPN patients received approximately 88% of the idealized cumulative chemotherapy dose, and the dose at the 25th percentile was approximately 71%. Patients receiving conventional oral nutrition were able to receive approximately 84% of the idealized dose, and the 25th percentile dose in the control group was approximately 78%.

Of patients who were malnourished at the inception of the study, those receiving TPN were able to tolerate 86% of the idealized dose; patients in this category and receiving conventional oral nutrition were able to receive 81% of the idealized dose. Again, this result was not statistically significant. Patients receiving TPN who achieved a complete remission were able to tolerate 89% of the idealized dose, compared to 85% for patients achieving complete remission who had received conventional oral nutrition. Thus, in this randomized, prospectively controlled trial involving adult patients with diffuse lymphomas, there is no evidence that drug tolerance has been improved as a consequence of TPN. Moreover, there was no significant difference in survival between patients recieving TPN or oral nutrition, whether or not the patients were initially malnourished. All patients have been followed until death or for at least 5 years following completion of therapy (recurrences after 5 disease-free years are very rare).

The results of this prospectively randomized study in adults with diffuse non-Hodgkin's lymphoma fail to demonstrate that nutritional intervention in the form of total parenteral nutrition permits a greater dose or dose rate of primary tumor treatment to be delivered. Therefore, there is no reason to expect that the TPN group would demonstrate an improved tumor response and longer median survival. Patients receiving TPN did gain more weight than patients receiving conventional oral nutrition. However, despite the fact that the maximum nutritional support permitted by currently available technology was administered, nitrogen balance was never entirely restored, and there were no significant differences in total serum proteins nor in recovery from bone marrow suppression between control and hyperalimented patients. Thus, idealized nutrition was not achieved with TPN in these lymphoma patients, although weight was gained and nitrogen balance was improved. The TPN regimen described here provided adequate calories, but did not necessarily test the notion of hypernutrition, i.e., providing an excess of calories for growth and restoration of tissues rather than mere maintenance.

Although such excellent tumor response results were not anticipated at the onset of this trial, the fact that the overall complete remission rate in this study improved to 72%, and the number of patients cured of their disease to approximately 60%, with or without TPN, indicates that the majority of adults with this disease now experience complete remission of the disease with readily tolerable chemotherapy regimens. Therefore, one would anticipate being able to demonstrate, at best, only a small influence of TPN in the treatment of this disease. Thus, non-Hodgkin's lymphoma, employed as a model for testing whether TPN can permit a greater dose and/or dose rate, now appears to be limited by the fact that patients can tolerate a relatively high dose and dose rate without TPN. Even higher doses may well produce more morbidity and mortality from side-effects that cannot be salvaged with nutritional intervention (e.g., heart failure). It is also possible that NHL patients not having a durable remission with ProMACE-MOPP are resistant to any dose of these agents. Moreover, the notion of hypernutrition, as opposed to the maintenance of nutrition, could not be tested because it is not technically possible with current methods. Nonetheless, TPN certainly did produce some nutritional improvement in these patients, but this improvement was not enough to make a difference in the rate of marrow recovery or any other event that would have permitted a differential in the dose and/or dose rate of therapy. Finally, since this disease is now so responsive to tolerable chemotherapeutic regimens, even hypernutrition, were it technically possible, would not permit a much greater intensification of treatment without compromising the already excellent response rates due to additional drug-induced morbity and mortality. It is of course possible that a small benefit with regard to improved dose rate and a consequently improved survival has occurred in this trial, but cannot be discriminated statistically due to our modest sample size. If that is the case, a very much larger trial would be required for proof of this small benefit—a benefit so predictably modest as not to warrant an expanded trial in NHL.

NCI TRIAL OF TPN IN YOUNG PATIENTS WITH POOR-PROGNOSIS SARCOMAS

A second prospectively randomized trial of TPN at the NCI involves young patients with metastatic or recurrent sarcomas (Shamberger, Pizzo, Goodgame, Lowry, Maher, Wesley, & Brennan, 1983). In contrast to lymphomas, sarcomas are notoriously unresponsive to chemotherapy in this setting, but there is still some evidence for a linear dose-response relationship. The tumors under study include Ewing's sarcoma, rhabdomyosarcoma, and osteosarcoma. The period of study in this trial involves one very intensive course of chemotherapy, or chemotherapy plus radiotherapy. Patients are randomly allocated to receive TPN or conventional oral nutrition during the course of intensive cancer treatment. Patients randomly allocated to the TPN group receive 40 kcal/kg/day (with nitrogen, 0.3 g/kg ideal weight) as a mixture of 20–25% dextrose and 4.25% Freamine. TPN is administered until oral intake is established at greater than 2000 kcal/day. At the time of this report, 12 patients have been randomized to receive TPN and 15 patients to receive conventional oral nutrition.

In this study, Ewing's sarcoma patients are enrolled who have either metastatic disease at presentation or a central axis primary tumor. In both settings, survival has been extremely poor. These patients are initially treated with radiation to all areas of bulky disease and with vincristine, actinomycin D, and cyclophosphamide. The patient's bone marrow is harvested and frozen, to be later re-infused in an attempt to "rescue" treatment-induced marrow suppression. The patient is next treated with a course of total-body irradiation (150 rads) followed by high-dose chemotherapy with vincristine, Adriamycin, cyclophosphamide, and DTIC. Marrow reconstitution with the patient's own frozen marrow is then attempted in a subset of the patients (Glaubiger, Tepper, & Makuch, 1982). The period of observation for the TPN trial consists of the total-body irradiation-high-dose chemotherapy-marrow rescue cycle.

Rhabdomyosarcoma patients entering this TPN study are those with metastatic disease at presentation or with disease recurrence. These patients are treated with cycles of DTIC, Adriamycin, and cyclophosphamide; with each successive cycle, the cumulative dose of cyclophosphamide is escalated (from one to four consecutive days of treatment). It is during the final cycle, during which patients may also receive marrow reconstitution and be isolated within special germ-free rooms, that TPN is studied.

The osteosarcoma patients in this TPN trial differ from patients with the other two tumors in that they have no clinically detectable disease. These are patients who either have presented with metastases or have developed metastases subsequent to diagnosis and the inception of adjuvant therapy. They have had metastasectomy and are free of detectable disease at the time of entry into the TPN trial. One intensive course of chemotherapy is given following metastasectomy, consisting of high-dose methotrexate, Adriamycin, cyclophosphamide, DTIC, L-phenylalanine mustard, and cis-platinum. Maximum tolerable doses of each of the drugs are administered.

In examining pre and posttreatment nutritional parameters in the two groups of the study, it was found that patients receiving TPN had a slightly lower preillness weight than did those in the control group. Mean caloric intake in the TPN group was more than twice that in the control group, and mean intake of nitrogen was almost six-fold greater among TPN patients. Nitrogen balance was much less negative in the TPN group than in the control group, but it is clear that even in the TPN group nitrogen balance was not restored. A least-squares linear regression analysis suggests that a caloric intake of 1875 calories/sq m (body surface area)/day and a nitrogen intake of 10.1 g/sq m/day would be required in this patient group to achieve nitrogen balance, but delivery of these quantities is limited by the necessary amount of fluid. The data demonstrate that there were no significant differences between the two treatment groups with respect to total serum proteins, or recovery from marrow suppression, before or after the period of nutritional intervention. Moreover, there was no difference in the frequency of clinical infections. As in other reported studies of TPN (Brennan, 1981, 1982; Copeland et al., 1979; Costa & Donaldson, 1979), there was a significant impact of nutritional intervention on weight, with 75% of the patients in the control group experiencing a weight loss and 90% of the patients in the TPN group experiencing a weight gain.

In this study of the utility of nutritional intervention in the treatment of resistant sarcomas, the proportion of patients demonstrating partial plus complete responses to the intensive course of chemo- and radiotherapy, and the median long-term survival, have not differed between the two treatment groups (at this time, the median follow-up is three years). With respect to short-term survival, patients in the TPN group do appear to demonstrate a small advantage (approximately 10%). However, a number of variables might explain this result, including germ-free isolation and autologous marrow re-infusions, as well as the prognostic implications of the particular but varied tumor types under study and their intrinsic biology and treatment. The two groups were roughly comparable in all of these variables, but with this small sample size, it is not possible to determine whether the apparent improvement in short-term survival of TPN patients is in fact a function of TPN or of the other variable factors in this group. Importantly, the results demonstrate that ultimately patients receiving TPN have not had an improved long-term survival as compared with patients in the control group.

The goal in this study was not to determine whether we could escalate therapy differentially between the two groups but rather, after the fact, whether tumor response was improved and survival greater because of less morbidity and mortality in the TPN group. However, it is now apparent that metastatic sarcomas in young patients, already resistant to initial therapeutic attempts, have such a low probability of durable response to any current therapeutic regimen that no matter how much tolerance to the therapy might be improved by TPN, the therapy itself may not be significantly effective regardless of the dose delivered. Thus, the NCI sarcoma study, like the lymphoma study, does not allow us to draw definitive conclusions—but for different reasons.

Although the two NCI studies were prospectively randomized and were undertaken in disease models that seemed appropriate at the time of the trials' inception, it is now apparent that factors are associated with both models that prevent definitive conclusions. There remains the question of whether similar, but much larger, trials would reveal a small influence of TPN on promoting durable survival.

In this regard, a large, prospectively randomized national trial of TPN in adults with small-cell lung cancer has recently been concluded, and more than 100 patients are evaluable (W. Evans, G. Clamon, and R. Weiner, in preparation). This tumor is responsive to chemotherapy but responses are brief; higher doses might improve response duration as well as the frequency of response. In this trial, TPN was given for the first two cycles of chemotherapy and radiation therapy. TPN given intensively over this 30-day period has not altered the nutritional indices during the subsequent year. Moreover, the marrow status was not improved by TPN, so the doses of therapy that could be given safely did not differ in the two groups of the trial. As might be anticipated, there were no differences in the remission rate or in the duration of relapse-free survival. It is possible that TPN given for longer than 30 days might yield a benefit, but the results of the three randomized trials described here, taken together, make it unlikely that nutritional intervention will materially improve the outcome of cancer treatment.

CONCLUSIONS

Following introduction of the concept of TPN support (Copeland et al., 1979), several small series of patients with malignant diseases in which TPN was employed were reported; these series involved both adults (Brennan, 1981, 1982; Copeland et al., 1979; Costa & Donaldson, 1979) and children (Hays et al., 1983). Weight was gained; the rate of recovery from chemotherapy-induced granulocytopenia was reported to be accelerated; and response rates to chemotherapy appeared, at least in some trials, to increase when employing TPN regimens. In other studies, immunological function was believed to have been improved by TPN (Hays et al., 1983). Moreover, patients appeared to have been protected from infections by TPN during the course of marrow suppression. However, a number of other reports noted the failure of nutritional support to influence the course of cancer treatment. In a study of adults with lung cancer, no improvement was found either in nutritional status or in survival. In a study of children with various tumors, no benefit from TPN was apparent with respect to tolerance to chemotherapy (Hays et al., 1983).

As already noted, the majority of these studies did not employ concurrently randomized control patients, but because the impact of TPN on ultimate survival may be modest, and because of the number of potentially confounding variables in the complex clinical setting of cancer and its therapy, it is evident that the value of TPN will only be demonstrated or refuted unequivocally in randomized studies among patients whose tumors reflect a steep dose–response curve.

The results of the two prospectively randomized NCI studies, one in adult patients with diffuse non-Hodgkin's lymphoma and the second in young patients with poor-prognosis sarcomas, failed to demonstrate that nutritional intervention in the form of total parenteral nutrition has permitted a greater dose or dose rate of primary tumor treatment to be delivered with the consequence of an improved tumor response and longer median survival. In both studies, patients receiving TPN did gain more weight than patients receiving conventional oral nutrition. However, despite the fact that the maximum nutritional support permitted by currently available technology was administered, nitrogen balance was never restored completely, and there were no significant differences in total serum proteins, albumin, transferrin, or recovery from marrow-suppression between control patients and those receiving TPN. While idealized nutrition was not achieved with TPN, it does seem likely that a sufficient nutritional improvement was obtained, such that any large impact on tumor outcome would have been detected. One may conclude, therefore, that the limiting factor in these two trials has not been nutritional status but rather the intrinsic biology of the tumors and the limitations of their response to available tumor therapy. This, of course, has been the limitation with other supportive care maneuvers. Supportive care, whatever the modality used, can only permit a given tumor treatment to be delivered. If the tumor treatment is ineffective, or only modestly effective, there will be no effect of supportive care on ultimate survival. If, however, TPN does act modestly in improving patient tolerance to a modestly effective treatment, a very large randomized trial will be necessary to demonstrate this result.

In practice, these preliminary data suggest that a large randomized study may be difficult to conduct with young tumor patients, or any group of patients with an infrequently occurring type of cancer, because of insufficient patient accrual. It may in fact be impossible to identify a subset of the pediatric cancer population which has a tumor that demonstrates linear dose–response relations with extant therapy and which exists in sufficient numbers to permit the demonstration that this subset has its response compromised by reversible malnutrition. Some idea of the magnitude of the appropriate controlled clinical trial of TPN in pediatric cancer treatment can be obtained through the following reasoning: One might assume that the true success rate with respect to long-term survival in a given pediatric tumor is 50% and that TPN may improve this survival figure to 70% (on the basis of nutritional intervention permitting a higher dose or dose rate of treatment). To demonstrate this 20% improvement with statistical significance, it is required that there be approximately 100 evaluable patients in each group of a randomized, prospectively controlled trial (Simon, 1982). If in fact the improvement in median survival is only 10 to 15%, then 200 to 500 evaluable patients would be required in each group of the study. It is evident that few if any centers, or even national cooperative groups, would be able to complete such a trial because of the relative rarity of pediatric cancer and the rapidity with which tumor therapy regimens change.

Although the two clinical trials reported here from the National Cancer Institute satisfy the requirement of a prospectively controlled randomized study design, the studies still have flaws which preclude definitive conclusions. For example, because the majority of adults with diffuse histiocytic lymphoma demonstrate complete remission of their disease with readily tolerable chemotherapy regimens, one would anticipate being able to demonstrate only a small influence from TPN in this disease. As earlier noted, one would require 100 evaluable patients in each arm of a randomized study to demonstrate a statistically significant effect, assuming a 20% improvement. Clearly then, the lymphoma results described here do not preclude the possibility of a modest benefit of TPN. Conversely, metastatic sarcomas in young patients, already resistant to initial therapeutic attempts, have such a low probability of durable response to any current therapeutic regimen that no matter how much tolerance to the therapy is improved by TPN, the therapy itself may not be significantly effective no matter the dose delivered. Thus, the NCI sarcoma study also does not allow us to draw definitive conclusions. Moreover, the patient population in the sarcoma study is not homogeneous in that there may be variables implicit in the diversity of sarcoma types studied which influence the therapeutic response in any given histologic type. The TPN regimens described here provide adequate calories, but they do not necessarily test the notion of hyper-nutrition, i.e., providing an excess of calories for growth and restoration of tissues rather than mere maintenance. However, in the trials reported here, the maximal nutritional support permitted by currently available technology was offered. Finally, although the majority of the patients in both studies had little caloric intake by mouth throughout the trials, no attempt was made to control oral caloric intake.

Thus, although the NCI trials have attempted to address the major methodologic problem in earlier studies of nutritional intervention during cancer treatment, i.e., the failure to undertake prospectively controlled, randomized studies in which TPN is the only variable, even the NCI studies preclude the drawing of definitive conclusions regarding a small benefit. Nonetheless, the NCI studies, together with the previously noted national trial in patients with small-cell lung cancer, do cover the spectrum of tumor responsiveness to intensive treatment: excellent, terrible, and good but not excellent. While one might speculate that even more effective nutritional support (''hypernutrition''), if technically possible, would better protect the marrow and permit the ''good but not excellent'' responses to become excellent, it seems to me that our results of the past six years demonstrate that the real issue is the efficacy of the primary tumor treatment, not the level of nutritional support. Moreover, more effective tumor therapy likely implies better drugs, not higher doses of the ones we have (except in very limited situations). Thus, the rationale of TPN as a support for ''steep dose-response curve'' therapy now seems less well founded than when the trials described here were first conceived. Certainly, TPN promotes a gain in weight (and possibly strength) in cancer patients, and may therefore improve the ''quality of life'' over the short-term. As a means to influence the outcome of cancer treatment *materially,* it now appears to be questionable indeed.

Finally, since this volume has a biobehavioral focus, it is well to remember the possible role of belief and conviction in the outcome of supportive care maneuvers. Clearly, a great many clinicians believe that nutritional intervention must be ''good''. Furthermore, the notion that nutritional intervention during cancer treatment should permit more therapy to be delivered (and that this should produce a better overall cancer treatment result) is so logically attractive that in the absence of rigorously controlled, prospectively randomized studies (sufficiently large to reach statistical significance), it is facile to accept the benefits of nutritional intervenion as an act of faith, particularly when encouraged by patients and families, for whom these notions—at an intuitive level—are at least as attractive as they are to oncologists.

REFERENCES

Brennan, M. F. (1981). Total parenteral nutrition in the management of the cancer patient. *Annual Reviews of Medicine, 32,* 233–243.

Brennan, M. F. (1982). Metabolic and surgical care of the young patient with cancer, including total parenteral nutrition. In A. S. Levine (Ed.), *Cancer in the young,* New York: Masson Publishing.

Copeland, E. M., Daly, J. M., Ota, D. M., & Dudrick, S. J. (1979). Nutrition, cancer, and intravenous hyperalimentation. *Cancer, 43,* 2108–2116.

Costa, G., & Donaldson, S. S. (1979). Current concepts in cancer: effects of cancer and cancer treatment on the nutrition of the host. *New England Journal of Medicine, 300,* 1471–1473.

Fisher, R. I., Devita, V. T., Hubbard, S. M., Brennan, M. F., Chabner, B. A., Simon, R., & Young, R. C. (1980). ProMACE-MOPP combination chemotherapy: Treatment of diffuse lymphomas. *Proceedings of the American Society of Clinical Oncology, 21,* 468.

Fisher, R. I., DeVita, V. T., Johnson, B. L., Simon, R., & Young, R. C. (1977). Prognostic factors for advanced diffuse histiocytic lymphoma following treatment with combination chemotherapy. *American Journal of Medicine, 63,* 177–182.

Glaubiger, D. L., Tepper, J., & Makuch, R. Ewing's Sarcoma. In A. S. Levine (Ed.), *Cancer in the young*. New York: Masson Publishing.

Goldie, J. E., & Coldman, A. J. (1979). A mathematical model for relating the drug sensitivity of tumors to their spontaneous mutation rate. *Cancer Treatment Reports, 63,* 1727–1733.

Hays, D. M., Merritt, R. J., White, L., Ashley, J., & Siegel, S. E. (1983). Effect of total parenteral nutrition on marrow recovery during induction therapy for acute nonlymphocytic leukemia in childhood. *Medical and Pediatric Oncology, 11,* 134–140.

Levine, A. S., & Deisseroth, A. B. (1978). Recent developments in the supportive therapy of acute myelogenous leukemia. *Cancer, 42,* 883–894.

Pizzo, P. A., & Levine, A. S. (1977). The utility of protected-environment regimens for the compromised host: A critical assessment. *Progress in Hematology, 10,* 311–332.

Popp, M. B., Fisher, R. I., Simon, R. M., & Brennan, M. F. (1981). A prospective randomized study of adjuvant parenteral nutrition in the treatment of diffuse lymphoma: I. Effect on drug tolerance. *Cancer Treatment Report, 65,* 129–135.

Popp, M. B., Fisher, R. I., Wesley, R., & Brennan, M. F. (1981). A prospective randomized study of adjuvant parenteral nutrition in the treatment of advanced diffuse lymphoma: Influence on survival. *Surgery, 90,* 195–204.

Rivlin, R. S., Shils, M. E., & Sherlock, P. (1983). Nutrition and cancer. *American Journal of Medicine, 75,* 843–854.

Shamberger, R. C., Pizzo, P. A., Goodgame, J. T., Jr., Lowry, S. F., Maher, M. M., Wesley, R. A., & Brennan, M. F. (1983). The effect of total parenteral nutrition (TPN) on chemotherapy-induced myelosuppression. *American Journal of Medicine, 74,* 40–48.

Simon, R. M. (1982). The design and analysis of clinical trials. In A. S. Levine (Ed.), *Cancer in the young*. New York: Masson Publishing.

Steiger, E., Oram-Smith, J., Miller, E., Kuo, L., & Vars, H. M. (1975). Effects of nutrition on tumor growth and tolerance to chemotherapy. *Journal of Surgical Research, 18,* 455–461.

12 Conditioned Nausea and Vomiting in Cancer Chemotherapy: Treatment Approaches

Thomas G. Burish
Vanderbilt University

William H. Redd
University of Illinois

Michael P. Carey
Vanderbilt University

If an animal is given food that is laced with a substance that later causes gastrointestinal distress, often that animal will develop an aversion to the food and, as a result, the animal will avoid eating that food in the future. This phenomenon is thought to represent a classically conditioned response which has evolved so that animals will select safe, healthy foods and avoid toxic substances. Although this type of conditioning, which is often referred to as a learned taste aversion, has been thoroughly documented by well controlled research (see, for example, Robertson & Garcia, this volume), few if any studies have taken the paradigm one step further and asked what would happen if an animal that had learned to avoid an emesis-producing substance were forced to ingest it? An answer is suggested by related research: If an animal is forced to enter a chamber in which it previously received electric shocks, the animal will often show many of the same behaviors that it exhibited previously in response to the shock, for example, urination, defecation, and frenzied movements, before any further shocks are delivered (e.g., Miller, 1951). That is, the animal will display *anticipatory* responses that have many of the same characteristics as the subsequent pain-induced responses. These anticipatory responses are thought to be learned through an associative process that is similar to the one that gives rise to learned taste aversions. A similar process might occur if an animal were forced to ingest a substance that it had learned would cause nausea and vomiting: Under such conditions the animal might vomit even before being forced to ingest the substance.

There may be little reason to be concerned with the outcome of forcing an animal to ingest a substance that it had learned would cause gastrointestinal upset, since this situation rarely happens in nature. From a human perspective, however, this topic is of tremendous importance. Every year thousands of cancer patients are given chemotherapy treatments that can cause a variety of adverse side effects, among the most severe of which are nausea and vomiting. Thus, cancer patients are encouraged—in order to prolong their lives—to take drugs known to cause severe gastrointestinal upset. As was discussed in detail by Redd, Burish, and Andrykowski (this volume), this often results in additional problems: At least 25% of these patients develop anticipatory nausea and vomiting; that is, patients experience nausea and vomiting even *before* they have received the anticancer drugs.

Anticipatory nausea and vomiting can be extremely aversive for the patient as well as for the medical staff who is trying to administer the treatment. In combination with the pharmacologically-induced nausea and vomiting, anticipatory symptoms can lead to or exacerbate a variety of nutritionally related deficits including anorexia, cachexia, and electrolyte imbalance (Dennis, 1983). For some patients these unpleasant side effects become so severe that the patients insist that their drug dosage be reduced, thereby lessening the chances that the treatment will have an optimal effect. A few patients have even refused further chemotherapy treatments, well aware that a hastened death is a probable consequence.

The purpose of this chapter is to discuss treatment approaches to the problem of conditioned nausea and vomiting resulting from cancer chemotherapy. The chapter is divided into four main sections. First, the treatment of conditioned nausea and vomiting by pharmacological means is discussed. The second section reviews behavioral treatments that have been used to ameliorate these problems in adult and pediatric patients. The third section focuses on important but unanswered questions regarding the development and practical implementation of effective treatment techniques, and recommends possible approaches to answering these questions. The final section provides a brief summary and a discussion of conclusions.

PHARMACOLOGICAL TREATMENT OF CONDITIONED SIDE EFFECTS

Antianxiety and antiemetic medications were the first treatments used to alleviate chemotherapy-related nausea and vomiting. For the most part, however, these pharmacological treatments have been used exclusively to control the nausea and vomiting caused directly by the chemotherapeutic drugs, not the nausea and vomiting resulting from the conditioning process. The effectiveness of these pharmacological agents in reducing nausea and vomiting has been limited. The early use of anticholenergic-antihistaminic drugs such as promethazine (Phenergan) and major tranquilizers such as prochlorperazine (Compazine) often provided little antiemetic benefit and frequently produced unwanted side effects such as drowsiness and lightheadedness (e.g., Frytak & Moertel, 1981; Laszlo & Lucas, 1981). More recent research on delta-9-tetrahydrocannabinol (THC), metoclopramide (Reglan), and dexamethasone (Decadron) has produced promising evidence for the efficacy of these drugs, although unwanted side effects or administration restrictions (e.g., the need for hospitalization) continue to limit their use by some types of patients. Readers interested in a more thorough discussion of the effectiveness of pharmacological agents in treating drug-produced (or unconditioned) nausea and vomiting are referred to recent reviews by Laszlo (1983) and Poster, Penta, and Bruno (1983).

While pharmacological agents have been prescribed primarily to control pharmacologically-induced nausea and vomiting, it is possible that they also affect conditioned nausea and vomiting for either or both of two reasons. First, pharmacological agents may directly reduce conditioned nausea and vomiting through their relaxing or mood altering properties, much the same as do the behavioral treatments that will be discussed later. The fact that antiemetics sometimes can completely eliminate postchemotherapy nausea and vomiting gives general support to this notion, because in most cases postchemotherapy nausa and vomiting probably results from both pharmacological and learned processes. Second, in accord with the laws of associative learning, antiemetic drugs will exert an effect on conditioned nausea and vomiting that is generally proportional to their effect on pharmacologically caused nausea and vomiting. The aversiveness of a conditioned side effect (e.g., its intensity and duration), at least when it first develops,[1] generally does not exceed the aversiveness of the corresponding unconditioned side effect. Thus, the initial conditioned nausea and vomiting will not be more aversive than the pharmacologically-induced nausea and vomiting. Therefore, if the early administration of antiemetic drugs were successful in limiting pharmacologic nausea and vomiting to very low levels, the aversiveness of any conditioned nausea and vomiting that might develop should also be mild. Of course, if a drug were found that completely blocked the development of pharmacologically-induced nausea and vomiting, conditioned nausea and vomiting would not develop. In conditioning terms, if an unconditioned stimulus is not introduced, a conditioned response cannot occur.

In summary, while pharmacological agents are used regularly to treat pharmacologically-produced nausea and vomiting, they are often of limited effectiveness, and they are prescribed almost exclusively with the intention of reducing the pharmacological or unlearned symptoms, not the conditioned symptoms. However, it is possible that these agents actually do reduce conditioned symp-

[1]Under some circumstances it is possible for conditioned responses to gain in intensity over time, even if the unconditioned response does not change or is never again introduced (e.g., chemotherapy were discontinued). This is sometimes referred to as an incubation effect.

toms, either directly through their pharmacological properties or indirectly through their effect on the strength and nature of the unconditioned nausea and vomiting. The routine prescription of antiemetic drugs prior to the chemotherapy treatment, and the development of more effective and less toxic antiemetic drugs, could contribute significantly to the reduction of conditioned nausea and vomiting.

BEHAVIORAL TREATMENTS OF CONDITIONED NAUSEA AND VOMITING

The absence of a nontoxic and completely effective antiemetic agent for the reduction of chemotherapy-related nausea and vomiting has encouraged researchers to explore the usefulness of behavioral strategies for the amelioration of these problems. In contrast to pharmacological agents, behavioral approaches have been used almost exclusively to treat conditioned nausea and vomiting and have not been applied with the aim of curtailing drug-induced side effects. When behavioral strategies are used to treat *anticipatory* nausea and vomiting, their effect on conditioned symptoms is straightforward since any nausea and vomiting appearing before the chemotherapy has begun cannot be pharmacologically induced. However, when behavioral treatments are used to reduce the nausea and vomiting that occur after the chemotherapy has been administered, they may be affecting pharmacologically-produced as well as conditioned symptoms. As with pharmacological treatments, therefore, behavioral treatments are explicitly aimed at ameliorating only one type of nausea and vomiting, but may actually affect both types.

Five different behavioral techniques have been used to reduce the conditioned side effects of cancer chemotherapy: progressive muscle relaxation training, hypnosis, systematic desensitization, biofeedback, and stress inoculation training. We focus here on the first three techniques because they are the ones on which well controlled, experimental data are available. Prior reviews of these three procedures (Burish & Carey, 1984; Redd & Andrykowski, 1982) have focused on the details of their designs, procedures, and effects. We cover these areas only briefly and instead focus on rationales underlying the use of these procedures in the cancer chemotherapy context. We then briefly review the research relevant to the remaining two techniques.

Progressive Muscle Relaxation Training

Progressive muscle relaxation training is a widely used general relaxation procedure that has been shown to be effective in reducing the stress-related symptoms associated with a variety of medical disorders and procedures, including hypertension (Shoemaker & Tasto, 1975), asthma (Moore, 1965), migraine headaches (Attfield & Peck, 1979), tension headaches (Cox, Freundlich, & Meyer, 1975), and preoperative distress (Aiken, 1972). Relaxation training can reduce muscle tension (EMG) levels throughout the body, reduce autonomic arousal, and lead to sensations of deep relaxation (e.g., Borkovec, Grayson, & Cooper, 1978; Borkovec & Sides, 1979). Although the original relaxation procedure developed by Jacobson (1938) took many hours to complete, recent adaptations of his technique appear to produce relaxation within 30 minutes (Bernstein & Borkovec, 1973). In order to deepen the effects of these briefer versions of relaxation training, and to promote cognitive relaxation as well as somatic relaxation, some investigators follow the relaxation exercises with several minutes of guided relaxation imagery in which patients are asked to think about very relaxing thoughts or scenes.

We originally speculated that progressive muscle relaxation training in combination with guided relaxation imagery would reduce the conditioned side effects of cancer chemotherapy for two reasons. First, we hypothesized that by focusing on the relaxation instructions and the feelings of muscle relaxation they produced, patients' attention would be diverted away from the sights, smells, and thoughts associated with chemotherapy treatment and on to relaxation-inducing alternatives. In effect, we hoped to reduce the conditioned responses by reducing patients' attention to and awareness of the conditioned stimuli. Second, we suspected that some of the gastrointestinal distress associated with cancer chemotherapy might be related to high levels of autonomic arousal and strong negative emotions such as anxiety and depression that also occur frequently in the chemotherapy context. By relaxing patients and having them focus on pleasant thoughts, we hoped to reduce their conditioned anxiety and depression, and suspected that this might have some effect on their nausea. We speculated that relaxation training could have benefits in addition to decreasing conditioned side effects. Many cancer patients complain of feelings of helplessness and lack of control in dealing with their disease and the side effects of treatment (Cohn, 1982; Holland, 1977; Meyerowitz, 1980). We believed that teaching patients a self-control procedure in which they could actively participate might increase feelings of control and produce a generally more positive psychological state. Also, relaxation training is easy to learn, relatively inexpensive, and has few, if any, negative side effects.

Three reports on the effectiveness of relaxation training plus guided relaxation imagery in reducing the adverse consequences of chemotherapy have been generated through our work with patients at Vanderbilt Medical Center. The first report (Burish & Lyles, 1979) was a single case study; the second investigation (Burish & Lyles, 1981) involved comparing a group of cancer patients who received relaxation training during chemotherapy to a group of cancer patients who did not receive relaxation training; and the third investigation (Lyles, Burish, Krozely, & Oldham, 1982) involved a comparison of a relaxation training group, a no intervention control group, and a therapist control group in which a therapist spent an amount of time with each patient equal to that spent with a matched patient in the relaxation training condition. The purpose of this latter condition was to control for any treatment effects that might be due to such "nonspecific" factors as therapist support and attention. The basic procedures used in each of the three investigations were similar. Patients with anticipatory nausea were studied across 5 to 11 consecutive chemotherapy treatments divided into baseline, treatment, and followup sessions. A variety of outcome measures were collected during each session. Pulse rate, blood pressure, anxiety, and depression were measured before and after the chemotherapy was administered. Ratings of the patients' nausea and anxiety during chemotherapy were made, both by the patient and the nurse who administered the chemotherapy. The nurse also recorded the number of times the patient vomited during chemotherapy. Finally, in the third study levels of nausea were recorded by each patient at home during the first 36 hours following chemotherapy.

In each study patients were first given a baseline session in which the chemotherapy was administered and the various dependent measures were collected, but no relaxation training was given. During the subsequent chemotherapy sessions, patients in the relaxation training conditions were trained in the use of relaxation and guided relaxation imagery beginning about 30 minutes prior to the chemotherapy treatment and continuing until the chemotherapy was completed. During the followup phase, patients in the relaxation training conditions used relaxation and imagery interventions on their own both before and during the chemotherapy treatments. During both the training and followup phases, these patients were also instructed to practice the relaxation and imagery exercises daily.

The results of the three studies have been consistent. First, patients in the relaxation training conditions, as compared to patients in the other conditions, reported feeling less anxious, depressed, and nauseated during and after chemotherapy, and showed lower pulse rates and systolic blood pressures. The nurses who administered the chemotherapy also rated the patients in the relaxation training conditions as being less anxious and nauseated than the control patients during chemotherapy. In the first study, in which there was not a control group, the same pattern of results was found by comparing the patients' and nurses' data from the training sessions to the corresponding data from the baseline session. Second, the results obtained during the training sessions generalized to the followup sessions, though the size of the treatment effects generally decreased somewhat during the followup phase. Finally, in the only study in which there was a therapist-control condition (i.e., Lyles et al., 1982), there were no consistent differences between patients in the therapist control condition and patients in the no treatment control condition, suggesting that the effects of relaxation training were not due to nonspecific factors such as positive expectancies and therapist attention.

In addition to the three empirical papers that Burish and his colleagues have published on the effectiveness of relaxation training, other investigators have reported single case or single group studies (Cotanch, 1983; Scott, Donahue, Mastrovito, & Hakes, 1983). The results of these other investigations have also indicated that relaxation training can reduce the distress of cancer chemotherapy patients.[2] In conclusion, the data generated to date strongly indicate that progressive muscle relaxation training, can be effective in reducing the negative affects, nausea, and vomiting that are often experienced by cancer chemotherapy patients.

Hypnosis

The use of hypnosis to reduce distress in cancer patients was suggested several years ago in the pain control literature (e.g., Hilgard & Hilgard, 1975) and many groups of investigators have reported clinical case studies on its use in the treatment of chemotherapy-induced nausea and vomiting (e.g., Dash, 1980; Dempster, Balson, & Whalen, 1976; Finkelstein & Greenleaf, 1982; Gardner, 1976; Gardner & Olness, 1981; LaBaw, Holton, Tewell, & Eccles, 1975; Olness, 1981). Unfortunately, none of these reports included objectively quantifiable indices of nausea, reliable observations of the cessation of anticipatory vomiting, or replication across patients. Two recently completed studies, one with a single subject (Ellenberg, Kellerman, Dash, Higgins, & Zeltzer, 1980) and the other with a single treatment group (Zeltzer, Kellerman, Ellenberg, & Dash, 1983), have provided somewhat clearer evidence of its effectiveness. In both studies adolescents were asked to report the frequency and intensity of chemotherapy-induced nausea, both before and after the use of hypnosis. Although patients generally reported that they received benefit from hypnosis, the lack of appropriate methodological controls rendered the results inconclusive. In the most recent study in this series, Zeltzer and LaBaron (1983) compared changes in severity of chemotherapy-induced nausea in children who received hypnosis versus children who received supportive counseling. Both groups showed improvement, but there were no significant differences between groups. In conclusion, although clinicians working with pediatric cancer patients are generally enthusiastic regarding the use of hypnosis to reduce treatment side effects, more rigorous research on the topic is needed before firm conclusions can be drawn.

Redd and his colleagues became interested in using hypnosis to control anticipatory side effects after having observed its effects in reducing pain in adults

[2]Kaempfer (1982) has also reported on the effectiveness of relaxation with five cancer patients. Kaempfer indicated that relaxation was not an effective intervention; however, sampling problems, a lack of objective data, and the uncontrolled nature of the study render these findings suspect.

receiving cancer treatment. In this research (Reeves, Redd, Minagawa, & Storm, 1983), 24 patients were given audiotape recordings of hypnotic inductions and were instructed to play the tapes in order to learn to induce self-relaxation. Most of the patients played the tapes in their hospital rooms, soon after receiving their chemotherapy. After a few days of training some patients spontaneously reported that when they played the hypnosis tapes their nausea as well as their pain was less severe; in these patients nausea was completely controlled. These patients reported that they could literally "turn-off" the nausea by inducing deep relaxation. Their skill was quite impressive: In the midst of vomiting they would visually focus on a point in the room, take a deep breath, induce relaxation, and immediately stop vomiting. Redd reasoned that if some patients could control *posttreatment* nausea and emesis, then it should be even easier for patients to control nonpharmacologically-induced, anticipatory side effects through the use of hypnosis. In order to test this hypothesis, Redd and his colleagues began to teach patients to block sensations of nausea in the same way they were taught to control their perceptions of pain.

Redd and his colleagues' research on hypnotic control of anticipatory side effects used an individual analysis, multiple baseline design (Redd, Andresen, & Minagawa, 1982). Six women treated with chemotherapy at the UCLA outpatient oncology clinic participated in the study. Each patient had been observed vomiting before the actual chemotherapy injection during a minimum of three consecutive sessions. Two outcome measures were employed in the study: nurses' observations of emesis, and patients' ratings of nausea.

Prior to its use during chemotherapy, hypnosis was practiced during two preliminary sessions. The first training session comprising visual fixation, muscular relaxation, and guided imagery lasted approximately 30 minutes. This session was recorded on audiotape and the patient was encouraged to listen to the tape daily in order to increase her responsiveness to hypnosis. The second session was held one week later using hypnosis procedures similar to those used during the first session. However, after the hypnotic procedure was begun the patient was led through the sequence of events leading to chemotherapy, including being transported by wheelchair to and from the treatment room.

The third meeting occurred in the psychologist's office on the day of the chemotherapy treatment. After collecting nausea ratings, the hypnosis procedures were initiated and the patient was taken by wheelchair to the treatment room for the chemotherapy injection. After chemotherapy the patient was taken back to the psychologist's office to be awakened from hypnosis. The patient then completed ratings of nausea experienced during and after chemotherapy.

This procedure was repeated during each chemotherapy treatment session until the patient had completed her prescribed chemotherapy protocol. The number of times patients were hypnotized prior to receiving the injection varied from three to five. For ethical reasons, analysis by reversal of treatment (withholding hypnosis during one chemotherapy session) was not planned. However, because of scheduling conflicts, three patients decided to undergo one chemotherapy treatment without the aid of hypnosis. The unplanned variation of procedures constituted a within-subject reversal.

The results of the study showed that hypnosis eliminated anticipatory emesis in all patients. Thus, the effectiveness of hypnosis was not related to the number of chemotherapy sessions in which patients had experienced anticipatory emesis or to when it was introduced during the course of a patient's chemotherapy experience. When hypnosis was not used (i.e., during "reversal" sessions), anticipatory emesis reappeared. When hypnosis was reintroduced during subsequent chemotherapy sessions, anticipatory emesis was again eliminated.

During the actual day chemotherapy was scheduled patients initially experienced increased nausea as the time of treatment neared. This trend drastically reversed when hypnosis was introduced. This effect was replicated across all patients on the 21 days when chemotherapy injections were administered with the aid of hypnosis. The patients' ratings of nausea also indicated they experienced little nausea when they were aroused immediately following chemotherapy.

In summary, there is a considerable literature on the use of hypnosis to reduce the conditioned nausea and vomiting associated with cancer chemotherapy. Anecdotal reports, case studies, and controlled investigations with differing levels of experimental rigor suggest that hypnosis can be effective in reducing the conditioned side effects experienced by many cancer chemotherapy patients. Moreover, these results seem to be independent of the type of hypnotic induction procedure used, whether it is the therapist-directed or self-directed, and whether the patients are adults, adolescents, or children.

Systematic Desensitization

Systematic desensitization is a counterconditioning procedure that is most commonly used to train phobic individuals to overcome their fears. The procedure involves three general steps. First, the patient is instructed in the use of a relaxation technique, usually progressive muscle relaxation training. Second, the patient and therapist construct a hierarchy of stimuli relevant to the feared situation, ranging from the least to the most anxiety-provoking. For example, in the chemotherapy context the hierarchy might contain various stimuli associated with the chemotherapy experience such as driving to the clinic, feeling the needle stick, etc. Third, the patient practices relaxation training while visualizing the increasingly aversive scenes/stimuli within the hierarchy (Wolpe, 1958). It is hypothesized that as a result of pairing these scenes/stimuli with relaxation, in the future they will elicit, in real life and not just in imagination, relaxation rather than fear or anxiety. With many types of fears, the data support this hypothesis (Wolpe, 1973). Systematic desensitization has been used in the chemotherapy context because it is hypothesized that the clinic stimuli, which are currently conditioned to elicit unwanted side effects such as nausea and vomiting, can also be counterconditioned to elicit an incompatible but preferable response, relaxation.

Three studies have investigated the effectiveness of systematic desensitization for conditioned nausea and/or vomiting associated with chemotherapy. Hoffman (1982–1983) and Hailey and White (1983) have reported positive anecdotal evidence from single-subject studies. Unfortunately, no objective data were presented in either case, making an evaluation of the effectiveness of systematic desensitization tenuous.

In a well-controlled study on the use of systematic desensitization, Morrow and Morrell (1982) randomly assigned 60 cancer patients to one of three conditions: (a) systematic desensitization, in which patients were taught an abbreviated form of relaxation training and while relaxed were asked to imagine chemotherapy-related stimuli (e.g., seeing the drugs, feeling the needle stick); (b) supportive counseling, intended to control for therapist attention, expectancy effects, and other nonspecific factors; and (c) no treatment control. Patients were asked to rate the frequency, severity, and duration of their prechemotherapy nausea and vomiting during two baseline and two followup chemotherapy treatments. Between chemotherapy treatments patients assigned to treatment groups received either two sessions of the systematic desensitization or of the counseling procedure. The results showed that during the two followup chemotherapy treatments, desensitized patients reported significantly less severe anticipatory nausea and vomiting and a significantly shorter duration of anticipatory nausea than patients in the other two conditions, who did not differ significantly from each other.

The results of the desensitization studies, particularly the Morrow and Morrell (1982) study, suggest two conclusions regarding this technique. First, systematic desensitization can be effective in reducing anticipatory nausea and vomiting. Moreover, these effects occur even though the desensitization procedure is administered at a time and place removed from the actual chemotherapy treatment. This point is important since it suggests that a therapist need not be present during actual chemotherapy treatments in order to teach patients to overcome their conditioned responses. Second, the benefits of systematic desensitization do not appear to be due solely to patient expectancy or therapist support, because patients in the counseling control condition did not show similar effects.

Other Behavioral Interventions

Biofeedback and stress inoculation training have also been used to reduce conditioned responses to chemotherapy, though neither procedure has yet been studied in the chemotherapy context using a well-controlled research design. Two reports have been published on the use of biofeedback procedures. Burish, Shartner, and Lyles (1981) used a case-study approach to investigate the effectiveness of a multiple-site EMG biofeedback procedure in combination with progressive muscle relaxation training. After three baseline chemotherapy sessions during which no behavioral intervention was administered, the patient underwent four chemotherapy sessions during which she received relaxation training plus EMG biofeedback administered before and during each chemotherapy infusion. Three followup sessions were then held during which the patient was asked to relax on her own during chemotherapy, that is, without therapist instruction or biofeedback. Results indicated that during and after each of the training and followup chemotherapy sessions, the patient showed reductions in physiological arousal (EMG, pulse rate, and blood pressure) and reported feeling less anxious and nauseated as compared to baseline levels. Weddington, Blindt, and McCracken (1983) described two case reports of the combined use of relaxation training and skin temperature biofeedback. Although the authors give few details about the procedures used and present few objective data, they claim that the combined biofeedback and relaxation training procedure was effective in reducing pre and postchemotherapy nausea and vomiting. The important question of whether biofeedback alone is effective in reducing conditioned responses to chemotherapy has not yet been investigated.

Moore and Altmaier (1981) reported on the efficacy of stress inoculation training with nine chemotherapy patients during a six-session training sequence. The general goal of stress inoculation training is to help people cope better with or "inoculate" themselves against stressors they expect routinely to encounter in their lives (Meichenbaum, 1977). Usually the patient is taught a relaxation technique, after which he/she is instructed to use this relaxation skill in anxiety-provoking situations. Initially the person is told to practice the skill during imaginary stressful situations, and gradually is encouraged to practice in the presence of the actual stressors. Moore and Altmaier applied the procedure to the stressors associated with cancer, including chemotherapy. Although no objective data were given, the authors reported that after the completion of stress inoculation training patients exhibited fewer anxiety-related behaviors including anticipatory nausea and vomiting. Additional research is clearly needed before conclusions can be drawn on the effectiveness of this broad-based coping technique in reducing the distress of cancer chemotherapy.

Summary

Behavioral techniques have been used for many years to reduce the aversiveness of chemotherapy, though it has only been recently that controlled investigations of behavioral procedures have been reported. These controlled studies, conducted independently by different investigators in different clinics using different patient samples, uniformly suggest that behavioral techniques can significantly reduce the aversiveness of cancer chemotherapy, especially conditioned responses such as nausea and vomiting. Moreover, since most patients in these studies had been receiving antiemetic medication before the behavioral treatment was initiated, the results of these studies suggest that the effects achieved with behavioral interventions extend beyond those that could be obtained by medication alone. Thus, behavioral techniques clearly appear to be effective, adjunctive treatments for many adult cancer chemotherapy patients.

IMPLEMENTING BEHAVIORAL TREATMENTS: ISSUES AND RECOMMENDATIONS

Although promising, the use of behavioral treatments for reducing the conditioned side effects of cancer chemotherapy is in its early stages. Several important questions concerning how to develop maximally effective and practical behavioral intervention programs have yet to be answered or, in some cases, even addressed.

Perhaps the most important question at present, from a clinical perspective, is how to make behavioral techniques practical for large scale application. Most hospitals and clinics across the country cannot afford to spend the extra two to six hours of professional time required for every cancer patient who has developed conditioned responses to his/her chemotherapy. There are at least three issues that are relevant to the development of cost-effective behavioral treatment programs.

First, research in noncancer areas suggests that professionally trained therapists may not be necessary for teaching most of the behavioral techniques that have been used successfully with cancer patients. For example, trained volunteers have been found to be as effective as professionals in the provision of many clinical services (see Berkowitz & Graziano, 1972, and Durlak, 1979 for reviews). Also, several studies (e.g., Davidson & Hiebert, 1971; Reinking & Kohl, 1975), as well as pilot data gathered in our clinic, suggest that audiotaped relaxation exercises can be effective in the reduction of physiological arousal if they are combined with limited therapist intervention and not simply given to a patient to use on his/her own. The use of lay volunteers such as family members and other patients, audiotapes, and similar nonprofessional resources may reduce considerably the professional time and expense heretofore associated with behavioral treatment packages.

Second, although the behavioral techniques described previously have generally been effective during the training sessions, their impact has often decreased during followup sessions when patients were asked to apply the techniques on their own. That is, often there does not appear to be an adequate "transfer of training" effect. For example, Redd et al. (1982) reported that anticipatory nausea and vomiting returned in each patient who missed her hypnosis treatment prior to a chemotherapy session, and Lyles et al. (1982) found that the effectiveness of relaxation training decreased in some patients during the followup sessions. While some researchers have found indications of transfer of training (e.g., Burish & Lyles, 1979; Morrow & Morrell, 1982), these studies have usually followed patients for four or fewer sessions. Thus, data are not available on chemotherapy sessions held beyond that point. Nonetheless, there is considerable practical importance to demonstrating a long-term transfer of training effect: unless patients can eventually learn to produce the treatment effect on their own, a therapist would be required to spend time with patients during all or most chemotherapy treatments. Although long-term transfer of training effects have not been documented with cancer patients, they have been produced in other contexts in which behavioral treatments such as relaxation training have been used (e.g., Borkovec et al., 1978; Miller, Murphy, & Miller 1978). A close examination of this research suggests that a more extended course of training, a more gradual transfer from therapist-directed to patient-directed relaxation, and/or allowing the patient to participate more actively in determining how to phase out therapist direction may result in considerably stronger transfer of training effects.

Third, existing behavioral techniques can be made more cost-effective if they are provided only to people who can benefit from them. Although behavioral procedures are effective for many cancer patients, they do not reduce conditioned responses for all patients. For example, Lyles et al. (1982) found that more patients in their relaxation training condition, as compared to their therapist control and no treatment control conditions, showed improvements across the various dependent variables, and that these improvements were generally larger in the relaxation training conditions than in the other conditions. However, as Table 12.1 indicates, there was a good deal of variance in the data, with some relaxation training patients showing no change or even deterioration on some measures. We have begun to investigate various individual difference factors that may enable clinicians to predict which patients are most and least likely to benefit from behavioral interventions. Preliminary data are encouraging in that there do appear to be factors that have predictive power. For example, consistent with data published elsewhere (e.g., Blanchard et al., 1982), cancer patients who reported experiencing very high levels of anxiety just prior to chemotherapy were significantly less likely to benefit from our behavioral interventions than were patients who had lower levels of anxiety (Carey & Burish, 1984). Patients with high levels of anxiety may be too aroused to attend to and comply with the behavioral self-control procedures, and as a result they may be less likely to benefit from these interventions. Results such as these suggest that individual difference factors may be very useful in predicting which patients are most likely to benefit from behavioral treatment efforts. Moreover, the identification of patients who are unlikely to benefit from the behavioral treatments used to date may lead to the development of alternate approaches for these patients.

Reducing therapists' time, promoting transfer of training, and identifying promising candidates for behavioral interventions should increase substantially

TABLE 12.1
Percentage of Patients Showing Changes of Various Magnitudes from Base to the Final Training Session on Postsession Systolic Blood Pressure, Anxiety Adjective Check List, Patient-Rated Nausea, and Nurse-Rated Anxiety[a]

Measure/Magnitude of Change	Condition		
	RT[b]	TC[c]	NTC[d]
Systolic Blood Pressure (mm Hg)			
Decreased 10 or more	50%	21%	36%
Decreased 1-9	36%	29%	12%
Increased 0-9	14%	29%	29%
Increased 10 or more	0%	21%	24%
Anxiety Adjective Check List			
Decreased 5 or more	36%	0%	22%
Decreased 1-4	43%	36%	17%
Increased 0-4	14%	43%	44%
Increased 5 or more	7%	21%	17%
Patient-Rated Nausea			
Decreased 3 or more	39%	7%	11%
Decreased 1-2	22%	7%	17%
Increased 0-2	33%	64%	61%
Increased 3 or more	6%	21%	11%
Nurse-Rated Nausea			
Decreased 3 or more	39%	0%	0%
Decreased 1-2	33%	7%	28%
Increased 0-2	28%	79%	67%
Increased 3 or more	0%	14%	6%

[a] Taken from Lyles et al. (1982), p. 521.
[b] RT = relaxation training
[c] TC = therapist control
[d] NTC = No treatment control

the cost-effectiveness of behavioral treatments. However, perhaps the most useful cost-effective approach is to focus on prevention rather than on treatment. It may be possible to prevent, delay the onset, or reduce the intensity of conditioned responses to chemotherapy. For example, the early introduction of behavioral techniques and/or pharmacological agents, perhaps even before chemotherapy treatments begin, may help to prevent or at least slow down the development of conditioned responses. Love, Nerenz, and Leventhal (1982) have suggested that for some patients certain tastes, for instance the metallic taste associated with some chemotherapy drugs, become conditioned stimuli for nausea and vomiting. Blocking or preventing the taste, perhaps by something as simple as sucking on a piece of candy, may help to prevent the conditioned taste aversion from developing. Also, research on a variety of other noxious medical procedures (e.g., Johnson & Leventhal, 1974; Wilson, 1981) convincingly indicates that anxiety, pain, and other symptoms can be substantially reduced if optimal preparation for the procedure is given. The most effective preparation procedures usually include giving information on the nature of the procedure (e.g., chemotherapy) and what it will feel like, sometimes through the use of audiovisual aids. It is conceivable that various interventions could be developed that would prevent or significantly interfere with the development of adverse conditioned responses to cancer chemotherapy.

Finally, it should be emphasized that the clinical effectiveness of behavioral interventions, be they administered to treat existing problems or to prevent the development of new ones, is determined in large part by the skill and sensitivity with which the interventions are administered. More than antiemetic drug therapies, behavioral treatments are interpersonal in nature, and the quality of this interaction can significantly influence the success of the intervention. In particular, we have found that two issues frequently emerge and can play an important role in determining outcome.

First, some patients believe that the use of a psychological or behavioral intervention implies that their problems are psychological in nature. This conclusion can appear to be reinforced if the person administering the intervention is a mental health professional. As a result of this reasoning, some patients become even more despondent because they believe the medical staff thinks that they have a "mental" problem. Other patients resist behavioral interventions because they believe there is nothing mentally wrong with them and therefore they do not need such interventions. We find it helpful to anticipate the occurrence of such reasoning, and to take steps to dismantle it from the very beginning of our work with a patient. For example, we discuss at length with a patient the normality of displaying conditioned responses to chemotherapy, and we explain in general terms how such responses develop and why behavioral techniques can be useful in reducing or eliminating them.

Second, a few patients are reluctant to devote the time and effort necessary to complete a behavioral intervention or to practice the technique at home. Attending to a therapist, listening to a biofeedback tone, creating visual scenes or images, tensing and relaxing muscles, etc. can seem very taxing to some cancer patients, especially to patients who tend to adopt a stoic acceptance of their condition or who have lost all confidence in their ability to help themselves. For some patients, practicing a behavioral relaxation technique at home serves as an additional reminder that they have cancer or that they will have to undergo further chemotherapy treatments. Our experience suggests that these concerns are voiced by a minority of patients, and that in most cases they can be successfully handled, especially if they are dealt with in an open and understanding way early in the course of the therapeutic interaction. Often we involve family members in the treatment process in order to gain their help in maximizing the patient's involvement, for example, by practicing the behavioral technique at home with the patient, or by giving encouragement to the patient.

SUMMARY AND CONCLUSIONS

Although chemotherapy can be a life-saving treatment for many cancer patients, it can also be a very aversive experience because of the many side effects it produces. Many patients describe intense and prolonged nausea and vomiting as the most severe side effects of their chemotherapy treatment. As has been amply discussed elsewhere in this book, most organisms develop learned aversions to gastrointestinally toxic substances, and as a result avoid ingesting them. However, since many cancer patients must undergo chemotherapy if they are to survive, they are in the unnatural situation of being forced to ingest substances known to cause severe gastrointestinal upset. The result for many patients is the development of conditioned responses that mimic the toxic effect of the drugs: nausea, vomiting, and associated emotional distress.

The first interventions used to reduce chemotherapy-related nausea and vomiting were antiemetic and antianxiety medications. These drugs have had little effect on anticipatory side effects, although it should be noted that they are usually not administered until the chemotherapy treatment has begun; therefore, their potential effect on anticipatory symptoms has not been adequately assessed. Within the last few years we and others have studied the effectiveness of behavioral relaxation procedures in reducing the conditioned side effects of cancer chemotherapy. Most of the data generated by these studies indicate that behavioral techniques can reduce the distress of cancer chemotherapy. This conclusion is remarkably robust considering that it has been generated by a number of research teams, working independently in a variety of settings, using uncontrolled as well as controlled experimental designs, and assessing outcome with a wide variety of self-reported, observer-reported, and physiological measures.

Although the behavioral data generated to date are positive, at this point they must be regarded practically as more promising than useful. The professional time and expense involved in most of the behavioral approaches investigated to date reduce the likelihood of their widespread adoption by time-conscious clinicians and hospital staff. Therefore, the next step is to modify these behavioral treatment packages so that they become increasingly cost-effective. Three potentially fruitful areas for research aimed at accomplishing this goal were identified. These areas involved modifying behavioral intervention procedures in order to (a) reduce the amount of therapist time required to administer the treatments; (b) increase transfer of training effects by teaching patients within a more explicit self-control paradigm; and (c) identify variables that will allow the prediction of which patients are most likely to benefit from specific interventions. Perhaps the most cost-effective use of behavioral techniques, however, will not involve treatment at all; rather, it may be one of prevention. Unfortunately, little research has been conducted on the question of whether behavioral techniques can play a role in preventing or delaying the development of conditioned responses. This may be one of the most fruitful areas for future investigation.

Finally, it should be emphasized that from the perspective of the cancer patient, conditioned responses to chemotherapy comprise only one aspect of what is a highly aversive situation. The pharmacologically caused, or unlearned, side effects of chemotherapy usually are as severe as or more severe than the conditioned responses, and behavioral techniques may have little effect on these symptoms. Thus, from a clinical perspective the use of behavioral procedures are not a panacea nor should they be the sole intervention approach to the side effects associated with chemotherapy. However, they can be highly effective against conditioned side effects, and thus we believe that behavioral interventions should play an increasingly important adjunctive role in the chemotherapeutic treatment of the cancer patient.

ACKNOWLEDGMENT

The writing of this chapter was supported in part by a grant from the National Cancer Institute (No. 25516). The authors thank Cobie Hendler and Michael Andrykowski for their helpful comments on an earlier draft of the chapter.

REFERENCES

Aiken, L. H. (1972). Systematic relaxation to reduce preoperative stress. *The Canadian Nurse, 68,* 38–42.

Alexander, A. B., & Smith, D. D. (1979). Clinical applications of EMG biofeedback. In R. J. Gatchel & K. P. Price (Eds.), *Clinical applications of biofeedback: Appraisal and status.* New York: Pergamon.

Attfield, M., & Peck, D. F. (1979). Temperature self-regulation and relaxation with migraine patients and normals. *Behaviour Research and Therapy, 7,* 591–595.

Berkowitz, B. P., & Graziano, A. M. (1972). Training parents as behavior therapists: A review. *Behaviour Research and Therapy, 10,* 297–317.

Bernstein, D. A., & Borkovec, T. D. (1973). *Progressive relaxation training: A manual for the helping professions.* Champaign, IL: Research Press.

Blanchard, E. B., Andrasik, F., Neff, D. F., Teders, S. J., Pallmeyer, T. P., Arena, J. G., Jurish, S. E., Saunders, N. L., Ahles, T. A., & Rodichok, L. D. (1982). Sequential comparisons of relaxation training and biofeedback in the treatment of three kinds of chronic headache, or, the machines may be necessary some of the time. *Behaviour Research and Therapy, 20,* 469–481.

Borkovec, T. D., Grayson, J. B., & Cooper, K. M. (1978). Treatment of general tension: Subjective and physiological effects of progressive relaxation. *Journal of Consulting and Clinical Psychology, 46,* 518–528.

Borkovec, T. D., & Sides, J. K. (1979). Critical procedural variables related to the physiological effects of relaxation: A review. *Behaviour Research and Therapy, 17,* 119–125.

Burish, T. G., & Carey, M. P. (1984). Conditioned responses to cancer chemotherapy: Etiology and treatment. In B. H. Fox & B. H. Newberry (Eds.), *Impact of psychoendocrine systems in cancer and immunity* (pp. 147–178). Toronto: C. J. Hogrefe.

Burish, T. G., & Lyles, J. N. (1979). Effectiveness of relaxation training in reducing the aversiveness of chemotherapy in the treatment of cancer. *Journal of Behavior Therapy and Experimental Psychiatry, 10,* 357–361.

Burish, T. G., & Lyles, J. N. (1981). Effectiveness of relaxation training in reducing adverse reactions to cancer chemotherapy. *Journal of Behavioral Medicine, 4,* 65–78.

Burish, T. G., Shartner, C. D., & Lyles, J. N. (1981). Effectiveness of multiple-site EMG biofeedback and relaxation in reducing the aversiveness of cancer chemotherapy. *Biofeedback and Self-Regulation, 6,* 523–535.

Carey, M. P., & Burish, T. G. (1984). *Anxiety as a predictor of behavioral therapy outcome for cancer chemotherapy patients.* Unpublished manuscript, Vanderbilt University, Nashville, TN.

Cohn, K. H. (1982). Chemotherapy from an insider's perspective. *Lancet, i,* 1006–1009.

Cotanch, P. H. (1983). Relaxation training for control of nausea and vomiting in patients receiving chemotherapy. *Cancer Nursing, 6,* 277–283.

Cox, D. J., Freundlich, A., & Meyer, R. G. (1975). Differential effectiveness of electromyographic feedback, verbal relaxation instructions, and medication placebo with tension headaches. *Journal of Consulting and Clinical Psychology, 43,* 892–898.

Dash, J. (1980). Hypnosis for symptom amelioration. In J. Kellerman (Ed.), *Psychological aspects of childhood cancer* (pp. 215–230). Springfield, IL: Charles C. Thomas.

Davidson, P. O., & Hiebert, S. F. (1971). Relaxation training, relaxation instruction, and repeated exposure to a stress or film. *Journal of Abnormal Psychology, 78,* 154–159.

Dempster, C. R., Balson, P., & Whalen, B. T. (1976). Supportive hypnotherapy during the radical treatment of malignancies. *International Journal of Clinical and Experimental Hypnosis, 24,* 1–9.

Dennis, V. W. (1983). Fluid and electrolyte changes after vomiting. In J. Laszlo (Ed.), *Antiemetics and cancer chemotherapy.* Baltimore: Williams & Wilkins.

Durlak, J. A. (1979). Comparative effectiveness of paraprofessionals and professional helpers. *Psychological Bulletin, 86,* 80–92.

Ellenberg, L., Kellerman, J., Dash, J., Higgins, G., & Zeltzer, L. (1980). Use of hypnosis for multiple symptoms in an adolescent girl with leukemia. *Journal of Adolescent Health Care, 1,* 132–136.

Finkelstein, S., & Greenleaf, M. (1982, October). *An hypnotic tape intervention for diminishing side-effects of chemo-therapy.* Paper presented at the annual meeting of the American Society of Clinical Hypnosis, Denver, CO.

Frytak, S., & Moertal, C. L. (1981). Management of nausea and vomiting in the cancer patient. *Journal of the American Medical Association, 245,* 393–396.

Gardner, G. G. (1976). Childhood, death, and human dignity: Hypnotherapy for David. *International Journal of Clinical and Experimental Hypnosis, 24,* 122–139.

Gardner, G. G., & Olness, K. (1981). *Hypnosis and hypnotherapy.* New York: Grune & Stratton.

Hailey, B. J., & White, J. G. (1983). Systematic desensitization for anticipatory nausea associated with chemotherapy. *Psychosomatics, 24,* 287–291.

Hilgard, E. R., & Hilgard, J. R. (1975). *Hypnosis in the relief of pain.* Los Altos, CA: Kaufman.

Hoffman, J. L. (1982–1983). Hypnotic desensitization for the management of anticipatory emesis in chemotherapy. *American Journal of Clinical Hypnosis, 25,* 173–176.

Holland, J. (1977). Psychological aspects of oncology. *Medical Clinics of North America, 61,* 737–748.

Jacobson, E. (1938). *Progressive relaxation.* Chicago: University of Chicago Press.

Johnson, J. E., & Leventhal, H. (1974). Effects of accurate expectations and behavioral instructions on reactions during a noxious medical examination. *Journal of Personality and Social Psychology, 29,* 710–718.

Kaempfer, S. H. (1982). Relaxation training reconsidered. *Oncology Nursing Forum, 9,* 15–18.

LaBaw, W., Holton, C., Tewell, K., & Eccles, D. (1975). The use of self-hypnosis by children with cancer. *American Journal of Clinical Hypnosis, 17,* 233–234.

Laszlo, J. (Ed.) (1983). *Antiemetics and cancer chemotherapy.* Baltimore: Williams & Wilkins.

Laszlo, J., & Lucas, V. S. (1981). Emesis as a critical problem in chemotherapy. *New England Journal of Medicine, 305,* 948–949.

Love, R. R., Nerenz, D. R., & Leventhal, H. (1982, April). *The development of anticipatory nausea during cancer chemotherapy.* Paper presented at the annual meeting of the American Society of Clinical Oncology, St. Louis, MO.

Lyles, J. N., Burish, T. G., Krozely, M. G., & Oldham, R. K. (1982). Efficacy of relaxation training and guided imagery in reducing the aversiveness of cancer chemotherapy. *Journal of Consulting and Clinical Psychology, 50,* 509–524.

Meichenbaum, D. (1977). *Cognitive behavior modification: An integrative approach.* New York: Plenum.

Meyerowitz, B. E. (1980). Psychosocial correlates of breast cancer and its treatments. *Psychological Bulletin, 87,* 108–131.

Miller, M. P., Murphy, P. J., & Miller, T. P. (1978). Comparison of electromyographic feedback and progressive relaxation training in treating circumscribed anxiety stress reactions. *Journal of Consulting and Clinical Psychology, 46,* 1291–1298.

Miller, N.E. (1951). Learnable drives and rewards. In S. S. Stevens (Ed.), *Handbook of experimental psychology.* New York: Wiley.

Moore, K., & Altmaier, E. M. (1981). Stress inoculation training with cancer patients. *Cancer Nursing, 4,* 389–393.

Moore, N. (1965). Behavior therapy in bronchial asthma: A controlled study. *Journal of Psychosomatic Research, 9,* 257–276.

Morrow, G. R., & Morrell, B. S. (1982). Behavioral treatment for the anticipatory nausea and vomiting induced by cancer chemotherapy. *New England Journal of Medicine, 307,* 1476–1480.

Olness, K. (1981). Imagery (self-hypnosis) as adjunct therapy in childhood cancer: Clinical experience with 25 patients. *American Journal of Pediatric Hematology/Oncology, 3,* 313–321.

Poster, D., Penta, J., & Bruno, S. (1983). The pharmacologic treatment of nausea and vomiting caused by cancer chemotherapy: A review. In J. Laszlo (Ed.), *Antiemetics and cancer chemotherapy* (pp. 53–92). Baltimore: Williams & Wilkins.

Redd, W. H., Andresen, G. V., & Minagawa, R. Y. (1982). Hypnotic control of anticipatory emesis in patients receiving cancer chemotherapy. *Journal of Consulting and Clinical Psychology, 50,* 14–19.

Redd, W. H., & Andrykowski, M. A. (1982). Behavioral intervention in cancer treatment: Controlling aversion reactions to chemotherapy. *Journal of Consulting and Clinical Psychology, 50,* 1018–1029.

Reeves, J. L., Redd, W. H., Minagawa, R. Y., & Storm, F. K. (1983). Hypnosis in the control of pain during hyperthermia treatment of cancer. In J. J. Bonica, U. Lindbland, & A. Iggo (Eds.), *Advances in pain research and therapy* (pp. 857–861). New York: Raven Press.

Reinking, R. H., & Kohl, M. L. (1975). Effects of various forms of relaxation training on physiological and self report measures of relaxation. *Journal of Consulting and Clinical Psychology, 43,* 595–600.

Scott, D. W., Donahue, D. C., Mastrovito, R. C., & Hakes, T. B. (1983). The antiemetic effect of clinical relaxation: Report of an exploratory pilot study. *Journal of Psychosocial Oncology, 1,* 71–84.

Shoemaker, J., & Tasto, D. (1975). Effects of muscle relaxation on blood pressure of essential hypertension. *Behaviour Research and Therapy, 13,* 29–43.

Weddington, W. W., Blindt, K. A., & McCracken, S. G. (1983). Relaxation training for anticipatory nausea associated with chemotherapy. *Psychosomatics, 24,* 281–282.

Wilson, J. F. (1981). Behavioral preparation for surgery: Benefit or harm? *Journal of Behavioral Medicine, 4,* 79–102.

Wolpe, J. (1958). *Psychotherapy by reciprocal inhibition.* Stanford: Stanford University Press.

Wolpe, J. (1973). *The practice of behavior therapy* (2nd ed.). New York: Pergamon.

Zeltzer, L., Kellerman, J., Ellenberg, L., & Dash, J. (1983). Hypnosis for reduction of vomiting associated with chemotherapy and disease in adolescents with cancer. *Journal of Adolescent Health Care, 4*, 77–84.

Zeltzer, L., & LeBaron, S. (1983, May). *The effectiveness of behavioral intervention for reducing nausea and vomiting in children and adolescents receiving chemotherapy*. Paper presented at the annual meeting of the American Psychiatric Association, New York.

Author Index

Italics denote pages with bibliographic information.

A

B

C

D

M

N

O

P

Q

R

X

Y

Z

Subject Index

H

K

L

M

N

O

P

R

S

T

For Product Safety Concerns and Information please contact our EU representative GPSR@taylorandfrancis.com
Taylor & Francis Verlag GmbH, Kaufingerstraße 24, 80331 München, Germany

www.ingramcontent.com/pod-product-compliance
Ingram Content Group UK Ltd.
Pitfield, Milton Keynes, MK11 3LW, UK
UKHW020939180425
457613UK00019B/467

* 9 7 8 0 3 6 7 6 2 1 2 7 8 *